Ayurvedic
Healing
for Women

Ayurvedic Healing *for* Women

Herbal Gynecology

Atreya

LOTUS PRESS

P.O. Box 325
Twin Lakes, WI 53181 USA

DISCLAIMER
The author, contributors and publisher can take no responsibility for the health and welfare of any person in using this book. This book is not intended to treat, diagnose or prescribe. The information contained herin is in no way to be considered as a substitute for your own inner guidance or consultation with a duly licensed health-care professional. We wish the best of health and welfare to all.

Library of Congress Cataloging-in-Publication Data

Atreya.
   Ayurvedic healing for women : a modern intrepretation of Ayurvedic gynecology / Atreya.
      p. cm.
   Includes bibliographical references and index.
   Formerly published under ISBN 1-15863-116-5 (paper : alk. paper)
   ISBN 978-0-9409-8595-7
   1. Women—Diseases—Alternative treatment. 2. Women—Health and hygiene—Alternative treatment. 3. Medicine, Ayurvedic. I. Title.
RA778.A8385 1999
615.5'3'082—dc21   99-11474
                                                              CIP

2nd US edition published by

Lotus Press, P.O. Box 325, Twin Lakes, WI 53181 USA
web: www.lotuspress.com
Email: lotuspress@lotuspress.com
800.824.6396

Printed in the United States of America

Dedicated to my mother,
Musette Elizabeth

who has continuously supported my study for the
betterment of myself and of all living beings.

And to the eternal, unmanifest Mother who
guides me in every thought and action.

Table of Contents

List of Figures

List of Tables

Foreword

I enjoyed reading this book very much as it matches what I experience with my patients. This book has a deep understanding concerning health in the sense that the root of illness is rooted in the mind. Symptoms arise from the way we live, eat, think, and behave.

Ayurvedic Healing for Women is suitable as an introduction to ayurvedic thinking and healing for beginners. It is also suitable as a study guide for advanced students interested in the specific health problems concerning women today. There is an underlying beneficial and optimistic attitude that trusts the healing power of nature and gives a hopeful outlook and comfort to most of women's problems.

The author doesn't hide the fact that there is a challenge for every woman to decide whether or not she wants to take responsibility for her own well-being. And this motivates us, as women, into stopping that inner habit of being a victim and neglecting our own resources. It helps us to face life consciously and joyfully—ayurvedically. This also means facing life as an individual.

In my fourteen years of working with and for women, I have found out that real improvement or healing only starts to happen when contact is made with them on a very personal and individual level—either physically, biochemically, emotionally, or mentally. The means are not as important as understanding the miracle of every divine being. With empathy, joy, and respect each individual person experiences a healing flow of energy—it's the life force.

Women today are not used to understanding themselves as a miracle and so tend to treat themselves (or let themselves be treated) rather mechanically, without the deeper knowledge of life.

To look at the wonder of life and trust the healing power in every single woman—that is what I have been taught by my patients and that is what I would like to hand over to other women, old or young. And this is what I think the book is a friendly guide to. I wish it a good journey throughout the world.

Elisabeth Hesse, MD
Basel, Switzerland

Introduction

Absolute Being, the One Queen, Transcendental
Goddess overwhelming the three states and hence is called Tripura.
Though she is undivided, whole, the universe
manifests in all its variety in Her.

—Tripura Rahasya

Throughout my childhood, I watched my mother fluctuate between a loving human being and an irrational person. This continued through much of her adult life until she had a hysterectomy in her 50s, at which point she stopped having drastic swings in her emotions and the chemistry of her body. She felt that a great burden had been removed. What was this burden and how was it created?

According to Ayurveda, any disruption, emotional or physical, in your monthly cycle indicates a metabolic imbalance; this is not a disease. This view is not recognized in the Western world by modern allopathic medicine or by society. In fact, the treatment that was given to my mother further imbalanced her and made her have broad emotional swings. The medication also created dependency. The social mores and conditionings molded her mind. These same influences reinforced the negative judgments of her children and husband. In short, what began as a sensitive nature and an imbalance in the chemical makeup of her body became a disease in the eyes of her doctors, her family, and society.

The medical community put her on hormone medication that apparently helped her in some ways for a period of time. Yet these same hormones further aggravated the imbalance over time, so that it became a chronic problem. These hormones also made her dependent metabolically. After a time, her body could not function without these pills. Still, she was troubled by drastic emotional swings, weight gain, and other problems associated with long-term use of synthetic hormones.

The sad reality is that modern medicine does not fully understand how to treat the hormone system of women or men. The scientific research community recognizes this and states so openly. Over half the women who begin hormone replacement therapy (HRT) stop before three months because of unwanted side effects. Yet doctors and the media continue to brainwash women that these chemicals are a preventive measure against heart disease and osteoporosis and that they will improve their quality of life. However, research studies do not support this approach, nor does the actual experience of many women. Their justification for these statements is based on statistical averages that change dramatically depending on the person doing the study and other variable factors. Unfortunately, this approach does support a whole industry.

This book is not "anti" anything, nor am I personally opposed to anything. I have used pharmaceutical products in the past and I may chose to do so again in the future. It is, however, critical in today's society that we look at the motivations of companies and persons in the medical and health industry. It is our health, after all. While your doctor may, in all good faith, be supplying you with information and a product that he or she believes to be therapeutic and safe, that may not be the case. While large pharmaceutical companies may have your health in mind, they most certainly do have their stockholders in mind. It is foolish to accept blindly a one-sided version of any medication or system of health. This book is about other options and sources of information. It is about increasing your knowledge. Knowledge brings power—personal power.

The oldest, continually practiced medical system in the world is Ayurveda. During the thousands of years of its existence, Ayurveda has always had a special branch of medicine just for women. This book endeavors to make accessible some of this information and to offer natural alternatives to women. It is only later in my life, after a great deal of study and years of treating women, that I have understood what happened to my mother. It is my hope that this information may save other women from the difficulties that troubled my mother. Her problems could have been corrected permanently in six to twelve months with Ayurvedic therapies.

Because of my own life—the family difficulties that arose from the medical treatment that my mother was given (women didn't have options or choices in the early sixties)—that I am writing this book. I feel somewhat strange writing this, because, at best, my knowledge can only be secondhand. I am a man. Yet, 85 percent of my clients are women and, through many years of being married, fathering a child, and practicing professionally, I have come to understand some of women's difficulties. However, it was not until I began to use the Ayurvedic system that I began to have consistently good results. I am clearly aware of the limitations of a man writing about women's health. *It is my hope that this book will inspire women practitioners to study Ayurveda more deeply in order to help women in all aspects of life.* Yet, the primary focus of this book is that of self-help for ordinary women.

Not all of the information in this book is traditional to Ayurveda. In the course of over twelve years of practicing natural medicine, I have gathered and integrated a considerable amount of information from other sources into the Ayurvedic model. This concept is not foreign to Ayurveda. The very name—Ayur Veda—justifies this approach.

Ayur is a Sanskrit word which is a synonym for life. It is also a synonym for the life-force, or *prana*. The one primary quality of prana is that it is always in movement. Life itself has one basic quality—it is never static. Otherwise, it is called death. Hence, the word *ayur* implies a changing and living system, one that embraces life, not one that reduces life to a category or fixed concept. Ayur signifies an all-inclusive approach to nature that honors and respects the most fundamental gift of being alive—change. Yet, it can encompass change and newness effortlessly, without losing anything. In fact, this change is a process of enrichment for the system as a whole.

Veda is another Sanskrit word which is a synonym for knowledge, in the sense of a logical progression, not a haphazard revelation of information. Veda is often translated as "science" because of this implication of logical, progressive development. Knowledge in this sense implies understanding. True understanding cannot be had intellectually or by study alone. Veda implies the kind of knowledge that comes from entering existentially into life itself. Understanding can only come from actual personal experience. Veda is that logical form of knowledge that comes from living and exploring the profoundness of life—of *ayur*.

Hence, one can see that Ayurveda is a living progressive system, not a dead or ancient method. The very fact that it has remained in use for over five thousand years attests to this fact.

You may sometimes hear negative things about Ayurveda, like the notion that women were isolated during menstruation because they were "polluted." These are misunderstandings stemming from the general rise of global male dominance and have little to do with the Ayurvedic system. The ancient Rishis, who developed Ayurveda, worshiped nature as feminine. They were very supportive of life (which is feminine) and so could not degrade woman or her body without degrading life itself. In Vedic times, women were given time to be alone during menstruation, not because of "toxins" but because it was understood that their attention and energy needed a brief time to turn inward. This is obvious in nature, where, during winter, the Earth's energy is turned inward. Because of this time of internalizing energy, spring is born. Women experience this cycle every month, reflecting the greater natural cycle.

Understanding this gave women time to nurture their creative potential, which many times manifested as the ultimate in human attainment, Self-Realization. The Rishis and their wives lived together in harmony and peace. Ayurveda is living in harmony with your nature and with life. Women today are not allowed a few days to turn their creative potential inward to its source. This is the cause of many social problems and personal frustrations—not to mention relationship problems.

This book is primarily concerned with treatments readily available in the West. Most of the medicines used in Ayurveda (in the West) are of plant origin. Therefore, I have used European and North American plant species for the treatments. I have used some other Asian plants that are readily available in the United States marketplace, as well. There are books already accessible that give apparently similar information. So why is this Ayurvedic perspective of value? Of what practical use is this book to women?

Ayurveda is by far the most effective system I have used. This alone is reason enough to look further into the system. However, the real benefit to women is that Ayurveda has a very unique understanding of the anatomy of a woman's body. This understanding encompasses, not only the physical and energetic body, but the emotions, the mind, and the spirit. It is this approach that could have saved my family from turmoil and eventual disintegration.

Ayurveda encompasses the biochemical model of allopathy (mechanical Western medicine), homeopathy, naturopathy, vibrational therapies, body work, and other subtle therapies. Yet none of these systems or methods can encompass Ayurveda. It is too vast. Ayurveda understands and, when appropriate, uses these other approaches. However, they are limited in view, according to the Ayurvedic understanding of life.

When I look for treatment, I first search for a system that treats me as an individual—one that honors me as a person. Ayurveda honors you as a person first and as a woman second. There is no one treatment for menstrual irregularities. The proper method depends on who you are and the context of your life.

Many holistic practitioners are now using this ancient approach of Ayurveda. Yet Ayurveda goes deeper. It is the only system that has a highly developed logical system to support its understanding of the different natures of individuals and, hence, their treatment. This is called the Tri-Dosha theory and forms the basis of the Ayurvedic system. Once you have used this system, its advantages become obvious. Tri-Dosha not only allows you to effectively choose the herbal remedies that are correct for you with much greater accuracy, it also allows you to structure your diet on a more profound level than the biochemical nutritional model.

For example a common plant that is recommended for many women, angelica (Angelica archangelica), has an action that improves blood circulation (among other things) and is therefore known to promote and regulate menstruation. However, when used according to Ayurvedic pharmacology, its use changes greatly according to the individual who is taking it. This is the major reason why different women get different results using the same plant. Ayurveda can give direction as to the exact use and varying effects of a plant.

This same reasoning also applies to dietary programs. Why does one diet program work for your friend and not for you? It takes very little observation to realize that we are all different types of individuals. Hence, any dietary, nutritional, or medical system that does not account for your uniqueness is, by its nature, limited. The exception to this occurs when you do not wish to be responsible for your own health, but give that responsibility—and power—to another individual in the medical community.

The wanton abdication of your personal power and dignity to the medical community (which encourages you to give over your responsibility), also occurs with respect to the commercial aspect of society. Women are a huge economic force in society. Women as a group are targeted and manipulated to constantly create new markets. One simple example of this was the introduction, in the mid-60s, of products for vaginal odor—a previously unknown "problem." Women were bombarded with advertising leading them to believe that they "needed" this product. From an Ayurvedic point of view, these products disrupt the natural balance that exists in the vagina and actually cause imbalances that can cause strong odor, vaginal infections, or urinary infections.

This is only one of many, many mass-marketing projects that reduce a woman's personal power and health. The best response to this reality in today's society is, not to become reactionary, but to rather become intelligent. Educate yourself to the many options that exist in natural medicine and treatments. Become alert to market manipulations and choose products because you like them, not because everyone else has or uses them. In health care, this trend is frightening. Be very careful in choosing a therapeutic treatment line and research carefully the known secondary effects. Then you must surmise the unknown or unpublished secondary effects by speaking with others. Often, these effects are small and subjective, which renders them all the more dangerous as your quality of life declines and your happiness disappears.

Knowledge is power. Personal power gives you responsibility for your own body. Without knowledge, how can you make an intelligent decision about your health? Why was the hysterectomy the most frequently performed operation in the United States for a decade? Can it really be that one-third of all women in the United States are so ill that they need to have their reproductive organs removed? Is it not more indicative that that particular operation was the most lucrative procedure for doctors and medical suppliers for a decade?

Recent publications in the *Journal of the American Medical Association* (Spring, 1998) have shown that over 100,000 people die in hospitals each year from the effects of *approved* pharmaceutical drugs. The study also points out that an additional two million people are left seriously ill because of approved medication. This study covered only the hospital use of drugs, not those in use by private medical practitioners. In contrast there have been no known deaths resulting from the *medicinal* use of plants in the United States for thirty years, according to the American Association of Poison Control Centers (AAPCC) and the Food and Drug Administration (FDA).[1]

Without knowledge, you have no power. Ayurveda provides knowledge, responsibility, personal power, and an easy, practical method of self-care. This book makes an effort to present an option to mechanical medical systems and also to add a deeper dimension to the "natural" forms of medicine. It also looks at the social role that conditions and dominates women and how they care for their bodies. Ayurveda, as a system, works first to correct basic metabolic imbalances so that symptoms can be addressed. "Natural" medicine that treats only the symptom is, in fact, still mechanical in its approach. This book endeavors to explain this information and empower you with knowledge.

The ultimate goal of Ayurveda is not health, but peace—in its greatest sense, peace of mind and peace in your soul. This is the goal of all humanity. Health will come when there is peace in the soul and in the mind, but health will not necessarily bring peace. Disease is seen in Ayurveda as a sign of discord in your soul and mind. Physical problems often result from this discord. Ayurveda helps you to find health on all levels. Peace is what Ayurveda can bring to women of all ages. If peace is not there, if happiness is not there, can health really exist?

Was the burden that my mother carried for much of her adult life a disease or a creation of society and the medical knowledge of the time? Tragically, it was a creation that relied on a complete lack of understanding by society and the medical profession of the time. This book will present, in a

---

[1] Herb Research Foundation, "Herb Safety Report," see Appendix 5 for more information.

clear manner, this case and show you how to prevent the same tragedy from happening to yourself or your loved ones. This book uses the Ayurvedic model to present a different point of view on health care for women. It is my professional experience that this methodology not only works, but works permanently and thoroughly, without side effects. It is supported by over five thousand years of clinical data and experience. It is a part of the science of life, Ayurveda.

PART ONE

Ayurveda and You

CHAPTER ONE

The Ayurvedic Perspective

That Devi Tripura, who is the conscious core
of the heart and therefore knows each one intimately,
swiftly rescues Her unswerving devotees from the jaws
of death, after manifesting Herself in their hearts.

—Tripura Rahasya

While looking through the many different books, articles, and studies of women's health, one becomes acutely aware of how many times the following phrase is used: "The exact origins of this disorder are not known." This sentence, or others similar to it, are reason enough to investigate the Ayurvedic perspective.

Ayurveda uses a much more profound approach to understand the functions of a woman's body than the material and psychological view popular today. Both the physical science of medicine and the mental science of psychiatry are ready to admit that there is much yet to learn in regard to the human being. This may be because the methodology used to understand humans is based on questionable grounds.

The Ayurvedic system is not a magic cure for all the troubles of humanity. It does, however, offer a completely different approach to nature than the system society presently endorses. In this view, Ayurveda offers a feminine approach to life and all that is contained within it. Ayurveda is an all-inclusive approach that is as unconditional as Mother Nature or the archetype of the Nature Goddess. Ayurveda has no condemnation of anything occurring in nature, for that would be a condemnation of herself.

Ayurveda is feminine in all aspects and manners of therapy. It uses all forms of known medical systems and all naturally occurring substances to treat all known forms of disease. Yet, always, its approach is unobtrusive and nonviolent. It never seeks to harm or invade another, but rather seeks harmony and peace by understanding the three great principles of the Nature Goddess—life, light, and love. These three are called the Tri-Dosha in the Ayurvedic system and represent the principles of movement, transformation, and cohesion on the manifest plain of existence.

As a reflection of the Divine Mother, Ayurvedic medecine cares for and nourishes without judgment or opinion, using the strict discipline of the loving mother to correct bad habits and teach habits that are in harmony with the greater workings of the universe. Yet, it is never invasive or aggressive. It may frighten and invigorate us through its power, may overwhelm us with its immensity and perfection. But most of all, Ayurveda will teach us peace and how to live in harmony with ourselves and others. This is the Ayurvedic perspective.

The wisdom of Ayurveda shows us the hidden causes, the subtle functionings of the body, mind, and soul. With this vision, the unity of life is revealed and the fragmented vision of mechanical times is put into its correct place as a servant, not a master, of life. In Ayuredic medicine, the Divine Mother reveals herself to those who approach her with love and the well-being of others in mind. In her own language, she reveals the source of disease. Ayurveda is her language. To understand her, we must learn something of how she functions.

CHAPTER TWO

You as an Individual Woman

*Then realizing the pure consciousness inhering as Self
to be that self-same Tripura, he became aware of the
One Self holding all, and was liberated.*

—Tripura Rahasya

The fundamental point of Ayurveda is that everything is interrelated. Nothing is separate in the universe or the human body. Another fundamental point is that the external universe is reflected in the internal universe of the human body. While everything is interrelated, each item is also unique. Each part contributes its own special quality to the whole, whether as a cell in the liver, as a human being on Earth, or as a star in the sky.

Hence, the concept of individuality is basic to the Ayurvedic system. Ayurveda only works with individuals. Yet, this understanding of the individual is within the context of the whole or Mother Nature. In Ayurveda, the word *Prakruti* means "Mother Nature"—that feminine quality that allows form to manifest. It literally means "nature," and encompasses the unique qualities of everything.

In order to use the Ayurvedic system, you need to have a basic understanding of how Ayurveda determines your individuality. In this sense, it does not mean to categorize you as a person. Rather, Ayurveda strives to understand how your organism functions, how your metabolism functions, how your mind functions.

This understanding of how our body and mind function is liberating. It frees us from society's stereotypes, from conditionings, from misconceptions and judgments we may have formed about ourselves. Ayurveda understands that each person is born with a basic nature that does not change. Understanding your natal or genetic makeup frees you from all the other concepts. This knowledge is empowering. Your natal nature, or constitution, is also called *prakruti* in Sanskrit. However, this is not the cosmic Mother Nature (also *Prakruti*), but the individualized nature. The word *prakruti*, as used in the rest of this book, will refer to the natal constitution of a person.

Ayurveda also understands that there is a changing nature or situation in the body. It is called *vikruti* in Sanskrit, which means "that which covers prakruti." This signifies a transient state of the body and mind. For example, if I have a cold, that is a transient imbalanced state. It does not indicate a change in my natal constitution, which remains fixed as diseases pass over it. The prakruti does not change during a lifetime. In very rare cases, chronic illnesses can change the prakruti and become the actual nature of the person. This is quite rare, however, and is usually terminal.

Once these two different states of the body are clearly understood, it is possible to proceed: our constitution does not change, but we are always in change. When our changing constitution (vikruti) is the same as our natal constitution (prakruti), health is present. When they are different, an imbalance is present. The imbalance can pass away with time, or it can become a "disease."

Ayurvedic theory is based on the assumption that, if you understand your natal constitution, you will take measures to prevent imbalance from developing in the first place. However, if an imbalance occurs, understanding your constitution can determine the kinds of therapeutic treatments that you should choose or receive.

Ayurveda also recognizes two different types of natal constitutions, physical and mental. The ancient texts say that these are usually the same. What many modern practitioners are finding today—especially in the West—is that this rule is not as fixed as it was in the past. We are now finding certain individuals that have different mental and physical constitutions. They are still a minority, but this can create confusion for a woman who is trying to diagnosis herself.

One of the main difficulties for untrained people is the confusion between the natal and changing constitutions. Often, clients of mine think that they are the disturbed state—usually a chronic situation—instead of their natal state, which they have forgotten over time. I will try to clarify the differences below so that you can identify your own natal state more easily.

Ayurveda determines your individuality by seeing which of the three natural forces dominate your organism. These three principles or forces were discovered by observing nature over hundreds of years. These three forces are not man-made, or theories, or concepts. They control the environment and all manifestation—whether we understand them or not. They are primal forces of Mother Nature, basically feminine in nature, and are not directly observable, although you can observe their functions and effects in the body and in nature.

These three forces are movement, transformation, and cohesion. Their names in Sanskrit are *vata* (that which moves), *pitta* (that which transforms), and *kapha* (that which binds). It is said that, to understand these three "humors" or forces, one needs to study them for eight years, as they are metaphors for Mother Nature's movements in the manifest world. These three principles combine to make ten different types of people. Seven types are traditionally recognized. For our purposes, however, ten types provide greater clarity. The main qualities of the three humors are given in Table 1 (see page 8).

Table 1. The Main Qualities of the Three Humors

Humor	Quality	Characteristic
Vata:	cold, dry, light, irregular, fast	(like wind)
Pitta:	hot, oily, light, penetrating, moving	(like fire)
Kapha:	cold, oily, heavy, regular, slow	(like water)

The humors combine in the following ways to make ten types:

vata	pitta/vata
pitta	pitta/kapha
kapha	kapha/vata
vata/pitta	kapha/pitta
vata/kapha	vata/pitta/kapha

There is more information on this subject in my book, *Practical Ayurveda*.[1] Ayurveda is a vast subject and any reading you do on it will be valuable. A very good book that covers this subject is called *Prakruti: Your Ayurvedic Constitution,* by Dr. Robert Svoboda.[2] The basic physical descriptions of the ten different combinations are:

1. **Vata:** Vata women are thin and either tall or short. They do not gain weight and have little or no fat tissue. Their arms and legs are quite thin. Their hair is dry, as is their skin. Their complexion may be darkish and they can tan well, though they may lose it rather quickly. They tend to have brown or dark eyes. Their circulation tends to be weak or variable, as is their immune system. Menstruation is often irregular, with little flow and sharp pain or cramps.

---

[1] Atreya, *Practical Ayurveda: Secrets of Physical, Sexual & Spiritual Health* (York Beach, ME: Samuel Weiser, 1998).

[2] Dr. Robert Svoboda, *Prakruti: Your Ayurvedic Constitution* (Albuquerque, NM: Geocom, 1989).

2. **Pitta:** Pitta women are of medium size and height. They usually do not gain much weight until age 36 to 39, and even then perhaps only a few pounds. They have a fair amount of fat tissue, enough to give form, but not too much. Their hair is slightly oily and may turn gray at a young age. Their skin is slightly oily and prone to infections or pimples, even later as an adult. Their complexion may be fair or reddish, in either case they sunburn easily. Their hair tends to be light colored and prone to dandruff. Their eyes are generally light in color, blue, green, or gray. Their circulation is good. Their immune system is normally good. Menstruation is often profuse, with dark-red blood, sometimes accompanied by pain. They can have a tendency to vaginal or urinary infections.

3. **Kapha:** Kapha women are larger than the other two types. They may be either taller or shorter, but they have thicker bones and bodies. They are physically the strongest. They can be normal or overweight in size. However, they always tend to put on weight easily and so must be aware their whole lives of eating habits. They tend to have thicker arms and legs than the other types. They have the best quality of skin and hair, both slightly oily, but with good luster. Their complexion is fair or whitish, yet they tan well and evenly and they hold their tans well. Their eyes can be of any color, though they tend to be brownish. Often, they have poor circulation. They have the strongest immune system. Menstruation is very regular, with medium flow, usually little or no pain. If pain is present, it is dull and achy. They are prone to accumulations that can result in fibroids and tumors.

4. **Vata/Pitta:** These women are usually less thin than the pure vata types, but can have a vata-type body. The skin gives a clear indication if pitta is present—it is oily and often prone to pimples or infections. The hair may be thin and dry (vata) or oily and with dandruff (pitta), or a mix of both. These indications will help you see if there is a

combination of both vata and pitta. Vata types have irregular circulation; pitta types have good circulation. These types tend to fluctuate between the two. Menstruation is irregular, sometimes with pain and irregular flows—sometimes heavy, sometimes light.

5. **Vata/Kapha:** These women have either a vata or a thinner kapha-type body. They tend to be shorter rather than taller. Usually, if vata is first they tend to have a more vata-type body. The skin is a good indication: is it oily or dry? Thinner with oily skin and no inflammations is a good indication of vata/kapha. V/K types tend to have poor circulation, with cold hands and feet. Menstruation is more regular and with less pain; flow is minimal or light.

6. **Pitta/Vata:** These women are fairer in complexion, perhaps still thin, yet with oilier skin and hair than V/P types. They are more prone to reddish skin and pimples. They burn more easily in the Sun. Menstruation tends to be heavier, with fewer irregularities, yet they are more prone to infections and irritations in the vagina.

7. **Pitta/Kapha:** These women are strong in body, with good muscles. They tend to be larger, but not necessarily fatter, than other pitta types. This is a very good constitution for athletics and sports (though exercise is good for all types). They may have a problem with oily hair or skin, and have occasional problems with inflammation. Their circulation is good. Menstruation is heavier rather than lighter, yet regular and with little or no pain. Sometimes infections can occur, such as yeast infections with mucous discharge.

8. **Kapha/Vata:** These women are larger than other dual types that include vata. They have good skin and hair. They may have pale skin. Vata tends to manifest as irregularities in the body or mind. They may occasionally have dry skin. Menstruation is regular, with light flow. Pain can occur at

times, as can blockages or accumulations such as fibroids and cysts.

9. **Kapha/Pitta:** These women are larger than other dual types with pitta. They are strong, if fit, and have great endurance. This mix gives them better circulation than pure kapha types. Menstruation is regular, with a heavier flow than a pure kapha type. Pain is generally absent, but the tendency toward infections, such as yeast infections, and accumulations is there.

10. **Vata/Pitta/Kapha:** Traditionally, this type is said to be rare and exhibits a perfect balance of the three humors. According to ancient texts, however, this may not be our modern definition of perfect beauty, as it tends to reflect a large, strong, lustrous body with a fair amount of padding. This type is rare, and I have only encountered one or two in many years of practice in Europe. They are said to be the strongest and have the most endurance of all types. Menstruation is balanced, with a light flow that causes no problems physically.

Each of the ten constitutions has different emotional and physical qualities, some positive, and some destructive and problematic. Here are the positive qualities of the different constitutions:

1. **Vata:** Vata is creativity; it is intuition. Vata is abstract and fluid, changeable and adaptable. Vata is present in all artists of every medium; it is inspiration. It provides flexibility and is social, though not necessarily in a profound way. Travel and movement are enriching. Several activities are needed and pursued with joy. When in balance, vata women have light and easy cycles, generally shorter in duration—24 to 27 days and lasting for 2–4 days. Pain is absent and so are emotional swings. Some fatigue may be present on the first day of menstruation. Life is abundant and joyous.

2. **Pitta:** Pitta is the energy of manifesting things. It is driven and motivated. The quest is very important, as is knowledge and understanding the nature of things. The inquiring mind is pitta in nature. Pitta is discrimination of the mind. Pitta women can impart their understanding to others and assist or aid people through their knowledge. They like to create things and put ideas into form. They are passionate and motivated. They are full of life and enjoy the interaction of life, yet need to remain independent. They need and seek responsibility. Their mind likes and needs to be stimulated through learning and seeking. Pitta is the energy to initiate things. When balanced, pitta women have regular cycles with a heavier flow than the other types. Yet pain and emotional swings are not present. Life is exciting and passionate. Their menstruation time is average, 3–5 days long.

3. **Kapha:** Kapha is the energy of cohesion. It binds and provides the quality of lubricating or of balance and stability. Kapha is the basis of the body and of the mind for all types, as it provides the needed stability. Hence, Kapha is the quality of stability, mentally and emotionally. Kapha women are the archetype of the Divine Mother and they radiate unconditional love. When balanced, kapha is devotion to the divine or to life itself. Love is the balancing quality in nature and kapha is that love in an impersonal sense. Kapha people move little (as in locations) and prefer to stay in a known environment. This allows their best qualities to overflow. They are the most reliable and least self-oriented of the three in a balanced state. They enjoy being and need to be with others and prefer a few deep relationships to many superficial ones. Family is very important and they love to create a family when secure. They are less concerned with intellectual pursuits than the others and prefer emotional relations with live beings—plants, animals, or people. When balanced, they have very regular and light menstruations with no pain or emotional swings. Life is full of love and abundance. Their menstruation is longest, 3–7 days.

4. **Vata/Pitta:** This combination generally makes a woman creative and able to manifest the creativity in a concrete form. That can be in the arts, in business, or any walk of life. This is a good combination for teachers. They are usually very fun, energetic, and like change. Their cycles tend to be regular, with normal flow.

5. **Vata/Kapha:** This combination generally makes a woman creative in a more stable or concrete way. This tendency may be more likely to manifest toward people or animals than toward abstract material forms. Great power of intuition lies here. An attraction to nature and all living things is present. The cycle for a V/K woman is regular, with light flow.

6. **Pitta/Vata:** This combination generally makes a woman more passionate toward life and the interests that she has. There will be the tendency to be a motivating force—in an energetic way—for those around her. This is also a good combination for teaching or helping others in any kind of pursuit, emotional, intellectual, or physical. Her cycle is regular, with a good flow.

7. **Pitta/Kapha:** This combination generally makes a woman motivated with life. She gets into life and lives it. She wants a home and family, yet she pursues different interests or careers. She has great capacity for work. Her cycle will be regular, with an even flow.

8. **Kapha/Vata:** This combination generally makes a woman alive and bubbly. Talkative, friendly, and social, this combination has the stamina to relate directly, deeply, and clearly with many people. She is caring and intuitive in her approach to others and perhaps enjoys organizing others or events. Management skills with people are there. Her cycles are regular and light.

9. **Kapha/Pitta:** This combination generally makes a woman powerful and strong. She has the ability to do whatever she wishes in life. Yet she tends to be more humanitarian than material in a balanced state. She is a strong benefic force in society. Her cycles are regular and of moderate flow.

10. **Vata/Pitta/Kapha:** This combination can make a woman the archetype of a goddess. She generally radiates love to others, yet she is strong and possesses great strength of will and brilliant intuitive abilities. She is regular and has a moderate menstrual flow.

Here are the destructive or problematic qualities of the different constitutions:

1. **Vata:** When imbalanced, vata brings depression, stress, fear, anxiety, and worry. Irregularities manifest throughout the body and the mind. All nervous disorders are due to vata. Menstruation becomes irregular, with sharp pains and cramps before and during the first days of menstruation. The pain can be debilitating. Depression is common before menstruation. Menstruation can stop under extreme stress or depression. Vaginal dryness is caused by an imbalance of vata. Fatigue is generally present before and after the beginning of menses.

2. **Pitta:** When imbalanced, pitta brings frustration, irritation, anger, manipulation, and jealousy. The heat of pitta brings all forms of infection and inflammation to the body and the mind. If left untreated it can burn the spirit. Menstruation becomes very heavy, with a lot of blood loss that can lead to anemia, fatigue, and energy loss. Pain can be present before menstruation, yet not sharp, as in vata. A woman can get frustrated, and angry with those around her before her menstruation begins. Once it starts, she feels a great relief, but may also feel quite tired.

3. **Kapha:** When imbalanced kapha creates huge emotional needs and feelings of a lack of love and security. Kapha types internalize their emotions and self-destruct through an accumulation of emotions. This may take the form of fat, tumors, fibroids, cysts, etc. Generally, they try to avoid expressing their feelings, which leads to destructive physical habits. Their cycle can become disrupted by strong emotions, though it will generally still be regular. They tend to suffer more emotionally, with large swings of guilt, unworthiness, and failure, accompanied by a basic feeling that no one loves them. There is a tendency to accumulate water before the menstruation begins. They may have sore breasts because of water retention. They tend to become stagnant and inert in mind and body. Through this, they lose their vitality.

4. **Vata/Pitta:** When imbalanced, this type becomes erratic in emotional behavior and tends toward strong outbursts of a passionate nature. They suffer from irregular menstruation and inflammations or infections. They tend to get sore breasts or nipples, though irregularly. Vaginal dryness can be common, especially latter in life. Pain can be present, changing from sharp to general, both before and during menstruation.

5. **Vata/Kapha:** When imbalanced, this type can become very depressed in a self-destructive way, internalizing the depression with a feeling of no self-worth or guilt. They may have outbursts, but overall, they tend to just feel badly with no real external cause. If left alone, they can feel dejected or worse. Yet, if they are with others, they feel inadequate. Their cycle is irregular and may stop if a deep depression sets in for some time. They may have excess mucus or discharges, according to their emotional state, which is irregular. Pain is migrating, deep, and dull.

6. **Pitta/Vata:** When imbalanced, this type can feel angry and irritable, and be prone to violent outbursts. They tend to blame others for everything and create mountains out of molehills. They are prone to infection and inflammation in the vagina or bladder. Infections can move around and be difficult to cure. They have irregular emotions and flow, although the number of days between cycles may be consistent. Pain, if present, is more general, with more just before and just after the start of menstruation. Depression may accompany the swings of anger or frustration.

7. **Pitta/Kapha:** When imbalanced, these women can feel irritable and frustrated. They have the tendency to internalize most of the emotions they feel, yet an occasional outburst is likely if someone or something provokes them. They are prone to yeast infections or other inflamed, infectious discharges. Their cycles are regular in time, but usually quite emotional and disturbed. They may have heavy flows.

8. **Kapha/Vata:** When imbalanced, these women usually experience self-negating feelings of unworthiness, accompanied by depression. Outbursts seldom happen, as everything is internalized, although a general feeling of neglect and lack of love can trigger strong emotions. There may be sore or painful breasts before menstruation. Excessive discharges are common. Their cycles tend to be regular, but with irregular flow. Migrating, dull pain is also common, either before or after the start of menstruation.

9. **Kapha/Pitta:** When imbalanced, this type may have internalized anger, which sometimes can be projected onto those around them. Generally, there is self-destructive behavior that is held within, as well as an accumulated frustration with life and/or love. Accumulation of water is common before the menstruation begins. Accumulative and inflammatory problems may occur frequently in the vagina. Their cycle is generally regular in days, but not in emotions or in flow, which tends to be heavy.

10.   **Vata/Pitta/Kapha:** When imbalanced, this type can demonstrate the problems of any of the three humors. As vata is the most unstable humor, it is generally the one causing irregularities of time or emotion. It can stop the flow of menses or cause any form of dryness and emotional depression. Pitta will cause inflammation and excessive flow accompanied by anger or frustration. Kapha will cause retention and accumulation of fluids or mucus through self-destructive or internalized emotions.

Note that, in a balanced state, any of the constitutional types have smooth and regular menstruation. Sometimes there can be fatigue on the first day or two of menses. Yet, when you look at the imbalanced states, you see that all of them can experience some kind of problem.

It should be understood that, according to Ayurveda, vata is the cause of most diseases in the body because of its unstable nature. However, this is even more true for reproductive and hormonal problems. *A disturbance of vata is present in all forms of menstrual, premenstrual, premenopausal and post-menopausal problems.* This is true even if you have no vata present in your constitution. Hence, the treatment of vata is included in every kind of corrective therapy.

Very often, menstrual problems are due solely to a transient factor (vikruti) like stress or shock. This imbalances the vata humor and causes problems, as is explained in the next chapter. *The point here is that you may be experiencing symptoms of a humor that is not dominant in your natal constitution.* The only sure way to know whether you are experiencing an imbalance of your natal constitution (prakruti) or of your changing constitution (vikruti) is to see a practitioner. This is especially true if you are of a dual type, because in that case it is more difficult to determine what your natal nature is.

There is one very helpful trick to help you recognize your natal constitution. Look at your tongue in a mirror. A very wide broad tongue is kapha in nature and a very narrow tongue is vata. A pitta tongue in not wider than the outer edges of the teeth—it is between the other two in width. The mixed constitutions are between the pure types; e.g., a pitta/kapha tongue will be broader than a pitta tongue and narrower than a kapha tongue. This is a simple, but very effective, way to know your natal constitution.

CHAPTER THREE

The Female Anatomy According to Ayurveda

*Even the most accomplished among men have fallen
into the habit of seeking pleasure from woman,
for all consider her the best hunting ground for delight.*

—Tripura Rahasya

The Ayurvedic perspective of the human body is quite unique. The insights that Ayurveda offers us are helpful, not only with diagnosis and treatment, but also with understanding the root causes of disease.

There is a perception in Ayurveda of the female anatomy that is especially useful in understanding many common problems associated with menstruation. Many of these elusive problems become clear when seen from the Ayurvedic point of view. This chapter attempts to provide a new insight into the female body.

It is interesting that Ayurvedic medicine did not have any moral problem with dissecting the human body prior to the rise of Buddhism around 400 B.C. In fact Ayurvedic medicine had the first medical university in the world and scholars from every civilization went there to learn. One of their specialties was surgery. Ancient doctors often had to treat people wounded in wars or in accidents. Thus Ayurveda is very familiar with the physical elements of the human body. In addition to the normal physical anatomy, however, which Ayurveda recognizes and uses, Ayurveda recognizes that the human body is comprised of more subtle components. Among these are:

three doshas (humors);
fifteen subdoshas (five subhumors for each primary humor);
seven dhatus (seven tissue levels of the body);
sixteen srotas (sixteen channels that carry both subtle or
    gross matter in the body);
seven kalas (seven membranes that separate the tissues from
    the channels).

The three main doshas and their various natal combinations
have already been discussed in the previous chapter. However, we have yet to look at their actual physical functions in
the body. Below there is a brief description of each main humor, and a description of the five subdoshas that actually
implement the general actions of the main humor. Each of
the subdoshas controls a function or system of the body.
These are useful for a woman to know because certain signs
can indicate which dosha is imbalanced more precisely than
other methods.

Vata (Vayu or Air)—In general, vata controls all movement
in the body and mind. It is the principle of movement in nature and in the body. Hence, it relates directly to the nervous system, which controls all movement. It relates to the
systems of circulation, respiration, muscular movement, motor function, the five senses, evacuation, lactation, menstruation, sexual function, and sweating. Vata is directly related
to the bones and bone structure. It creates dryness in the
body when too abundant and sluggishness when lacking. It
controls the sexual, reproductive, and growth hormonal
functions. The other two humors (doshas) are inert without
vata. The five subdivisions control the various aspects of this
general description.

    Prana Vayu: controls inhalation, the other four vayus,
the five senses, thinking, health, hormone function, and
proper growth. *Indications of imbalance*: emotional
swings, hormonal disturbance, low vitality, loss of senses, anxiety and worry, insomnia, emaciation, fainting,
disease in general.

Apana Vayu: controls elimination, sexual function, menstruation, hormone function, downward movements in the body, and disease in general. *Indications of imbalance*: cramps, pain, constipation, amenorrhea, dysmenorrhea, menstrual problems, PMS, hormone imbalance, dryness, urinary problems. Generally, all diseases are involved to some extent.

Samana Vayu: controls the movement of the digestive system, the solar plexus, and balances the other two main vayus, prana and apana. *Indications of imbalance*: indigestion, diarrhea, malabsorption of nutrients, dryness.

Udana Vayu: controls exhalation, speech, the upward movements in the body, growth as a child, and inspiration in life. *Indications of imbalance*: thyroid problems, problems of speech and the throat, weakness of will, general fatigue, lack of enthusiasm in life, disinterest in life.

Vyana Vayu: pervades the entire body as the nervous system, yet it also controls heart function and circulation of the blood. *Indications of imbalance*: problems of lactation, arthritis, nervousness, poor circulation, poor motor reflexes, problems of the joints, bone disorders, nervous disorders.

Pitta (Fire)—In general, pitta is responsible for all chemical and metabolic processes in the body. Pitta is the principle of transformation, on both a mental and physical level. Hence, pitta helps us to digest thoughts, feelings, and food—or transform them. Pitta controls all heat and heat disorders of the body. It controls the metabolic hormonal function. Pitta relates to the fiery organs in the body and the blood. It is carried by the blood in disturbed states. All inflammations are from excess pitta. Menstruation in general is pitta in nature, so any imbalance in menstruation has some relationship with pitta. Low pitta causes the whole metabolism to slow down and usually goes with high kapha. Excess pitta causes all kinds of burning and heat-related disorders, which usually burn up kapha and dry out vata. The five subdivisions control the various aspects of this general description.

Alochaka Pitta: controls the ability to see and the digestion of what we see and sense. *Indications of imbalance*: eye problems and difficulties in digesting what we see, mental imbalance, lack of discrimination, hormone imbalance.

Sadaka Pitta: controls functions of the heart, circulation, and metabolic hormones, as well as the digestion of thoughts and emotions. *Indications of imbalance*: heart failure, repressed emotions and feelings, excessive anger or unprocessed feelings, hormonal imbalance.

Pachaka Pitta: controls stomach digestion. *Indications of imbalance*: ulcers, heartburn, food cravings, indigestion, diarrhea, leukorrhea, candidiasis.

Ranjaka Pitta: controls liver and gall bladder, digestion, and blood. *Indications of imbalance*: anger, irritability, hostility, excessive bile, liver disorders, skin problems, toxic blood, anemia, menstrual problems (especially in excessive or diminished flow or menorrhagia), endrometriosis, cystitis, and PID.

Bhrajaka Pitta: controls metabolism of the skin. *Indications of imbalance*: all skin problems, acne, inflammation of the skin, vulvodynia.

Kapha (Water)—In general, kapha is responsible for the stability of the body and mind. Kapha is the principle of cohesion in the body and mind. It mainly exists in the body as plasma, muscle, and fat tissues. It provides the lubrication and basis for the body and controls flexibility and nourishment. Moisture and fluid retention is maintained by this dosha and all vaginal fluids are controlled by it. When kapha is too high, it restricts vata and subdues pitta. It creates congestion on all levels of the body. Too little kapha, like high vata, results in dryness and ungrounded thoughts and actions. The five subdivisions control the various aspects of this general description.

Tarpaka Kapha: controls fluids in the head, the sinuses, and cerebral fluids. *Indications of imbalance*: sinus problems, headaches, loss of smell, colds.

Bodhaka Kapha: controls taste and the cravings of taste, digestion, and saliva. *Indications of imbalance*: overeating and cravings for tastes, loss of taste, congestion in the throat and mouth areas.

Avalambaka Kapha: controls lubrication and the fluids around the heart, lungs, and upper back. *Indications of imbalance*: congestion in the lungs or heart, stiffness in the back and upper spine, lethargy, low energy, emotional stagnation, breast tumors or cysts.

Kledaka Kapha: controls the lubrication of the digestive process, maintains a balance with the pitta's bile, provides internal lubrication. *Indications of imbalance*: bloated stomach, slow or congested digestion, excess mucus, uterine tumors or cysts, leukorrhea.

Slesaka Kapha: controls the lubrication of the joints in the body and aids in all movements. *Indications of imbalance*: loose joints, swelling joints, stiff joints, painful movements.

The next part of the subtle anatomy consists of the different levels of the body. These levels are called *dhatus*, or tissue levels. It is simpler to perceive them as layers of the body, each layer giving nourishment to the next. In each level, the food and drink consumed by the body becomes more refined and nourishes each subsequent level in its turn. They also become more atomic or potent. The ultimate potency in the human body is the ability to create life. Thus, the reproductive fluids (ovum and sperm) are considered to be the highest, most refined, product of the body. They make up its seventh level.

The last level, or dhatu, also produces a substance known in Ayurveda as *ojas*. Ojas is the primal energy of the body and goes back through the cycle of the seven tissues to nourish all of its levels. Many modern Ayurvedic doctors who are trained in both allopathy (modern medicine) and Ayurveda, state that ojas represents our basic immunity. In other words, when ojas is low, our immune system is low. Ayurveda has a whole treatment method to strengthen ojas, and so our vitality. The concept of ojas is also directly related to fertility. According to Ayurveda, a strong, healthy seventh level and abundant ojas must exist in order for conception to occur and to produce a strong healthy child.

Each dhatu, or level has one or more sublevels as well. The seven main levels and their sublevels are shown in Table 2, below.

Table 2. The Seven Dhatus, Sublevels, and Waste Materials

Dhatu	Sublevel	Waste Materials
plasma and lymph fluids	mammary glands and fluids menstrual flow	mucus (the kapha dosha in general)
red blood cells (generally given as blood in general)	blood vessels muscle tendons	digestive bile (the pitta dosha in general)
muscles	skin ligaments	any accumulation in body cavities, i.e., navel, ear wax
fat and connective tissues	fatty tissue under skin	sweat
bones	teeth	nails, body hair
marrow and nerves	sclerotic fluid in the eyes hair on the head	tears
reproductive fluids	ojas (primary energy)	smegma (a discharge that accumulates under the foreskin of a male and can also accumulate between the labium major and minor of a woman)

Not only does each level nourish the next level and its sub-levels, it also has a specific waste product. The secondary levels and waste products are important because they can give us an indication of our health. They manifest as hair, nails, and body odor. A healthy level produces a healthy "waste." For example, if you have excessive mucous discharges, it indicates imbalances in the plasma level of the body.

The next part of the anatomy consists of channels, or systems. Some of the these systems relate to the Western view of anatomy, others do not. There are fourteen systems for men and sixteen for women. These *srotas*, or channels, nourish the seven dhatus, or tissues, of the body. They also nourish the organs and help to eliminate waste products from the body. They contain the dhatus that they nourish.

Some of these srotas are quite physical, others very subtle. Some exist as a fine web throughout the physical and subtle body; others carry the blood and food. These channels are indicative of good heath. When the flow through them is disrupted, disease results. They are disturbed by the three humors and the accumulation of toxins. Notice that the mind (especially the movement of thought) has its own channel. Ayurveda is intimately aware that the mind has a great effect on the other systems of the body and has never excluded this important aspect of the human being. The srotas are shared by men and women as follows:

Movement

Prana (Vayu) Channel: Prana is usually translated as "life-force." It has no real equivalent in English. It is called *chi* or *qi* in Asia. It is carried on the breath and is related to the respiratory, circulatory, and digestive systems. Another name for prana is vayu or vata. In this sense, it relates to the balanced or positive aspect of vata. It has no physical location. It is the *nadi* system in yoga.

Physical
Food Channel: carries the food and mainly corresponds to the gastrointestinal tract.

Water Channel: more than a channel, this is actually the whole water metabolism. It also governs the absorption of water in the body.

Dhatus
Plasma Channel: a huge network of canals that feeds the plasma dhatu (tissue).

Blood Channel: a large network that feeds the blood dhatu.

Muscle Channel: a large network that feeds the muscle dhatu.

Fat (Adipose Tissue) Channel: large network that feeds the fat dhatu.

Bone Channel: supports and feeds the skeletal structure and feeds the bone dhatu.

Bone Marrow and Nerve Channel: relates to the cerebro-spinal fluids that support the nervous system and feeds the marrow and nerve dhatu.

Reproductive Channel: relates to the reproductive and hormonal aspect of the uterus, and also is responsible for secretions during intercourse. It is related to the enjoyment of sexual activity; it feeds the reproductive dhatu.

Waste or Malas
Sweat Channel: removes toxins through the skin.

Feces Channel: removes unused or undigested food.

Urine Channel: removes unwanted liquid matter that the kidneys and liver have filtered.

Subtle
Mental Channel: relates to the physical aspect of the mind, not the higher aspects. It is related to mental disturbances that result from stress, physical shock, or trauma. It is primarily concerned with the movement of thought and the nervous system. Nervous disorders can find their origin here, as

the marrow and nerve channels are closely related to this channel. It has no physical location.

Women have these two srotas, in addition to the fourteen shared with men:

Menstruation Channel: carries the menstrual fluids and some other vaginal secretions.
Lactation Channel: dependent on the preceding system, governs the production and flow of breast milk. It also has a separate function with the breasts during sexual arousal.

Last, we have the seven kalas, or the membranes that separate the seven dhatus (tissue levels) from the srotas (channels) that support and feed them. They exist within the srotas and also protect the related tissue level from contamination or pollution. The kalas act as barriers and define the locations and roles of the tissues and channels. These membranes play an important role in the absorption and diffusion of nutrients throughout the body.

One of the most important kalas, for our purposes, is that which "contains" the bones *(purisha dhara kala)*. The bone and skeletal system is the main site of vata, after the colon. The health of the bones is directly related to the quality or balance of vata in the body. This membrane is actually the lining of the colon, the main site of vata.

When vata is disturbed, it accumulates and causes gas and toxins in the colon. However, when it is healthy, balanced and not accumulating, it produces prana. This prana is our life force—our basic vitality. This kala is responsible for the proper absorption of the prana from our food. *This form of prana nourishes our bones and prevents them from becoming brittle and losing mass.* When it is not functioning correctly, our vitality is lower, as is the overall health of our bone structure. I will explain this in more detail in chapter 11.

The above information will become more useful as we begin to understand how to treat the body according to

Ayurveda. In summary, the most fundamental aspect of the anatomy is the tri-dosha, or three humor, theory. These humors function through five subhumors. The humors move through the seven tissue levels, either nourishing them or accumulating and resting in them as disease. The tissue levels are the sites of disease. The normal health of the body is maintained by the seven tissue levels and they are supplied by the channels. These channels number more than the tissues and also support the organs and other mechanical functions of the body. The kalas, or membranes, act as protection to the tissues and also are *directly responsible for the absorption and diffusion of nutrients.* Health is the result of these systems functioning together in harmony. Disease is the disturbance of these systems due to a process that is described in the next chapter.

It is important to realize that you cannot use Ayurveda like a cookbook to maintain health and to heal. Unfortunately, there are books (along with practitioners) that describe a disease symptom and recommend a herbal recipe to correct it. *This is not Ayurveda!* This is a mechanical approach that simply uses plants or other Ayurvedic therapies to treat symptoms. Ayurveda is not a symptomatic system of medicine.

Ayurveda treats the root cause of disease through understanding the anatomy as described above. There is no cookbook that can be used with Ayurveda. Are you a fixed quantity? Do you want to receive the same treatment as every other woman? Haven't you tried this approach already and seen its limitations?

The treatment section of this book must thus be used only as a guide. It should be adjusted to fit your constitution and individual needs. The formulas are reflections of how I use the Ayurvedic system. The formulas in the case histories will show that I have adapted basic formulas to individuals. Often the formulas are quite different from the "basic" ones given for a disease or imbalance. This is not a contradiction. Rather it shows the need to adapt to the individual. Do not fall for the mechanical "cookbook" approach to Ayurveda and healing.

I feel that some basic points need to be made in regard to the Ayurvedic understanding of anatomy. The first and most important is that almost all hormonal imbalances or disturbances result from a deficiency in the seventh tissue level or *shukra*. Therefore, a woman must address the most subtle tissues of the body in treatment. As shukra is a function of the other six tissues, it is indicative of chronic tissue deficiencies. Shukra can also be affected by the mind, as can its by-product, ojas. Mental disturbances can "burn up" or deplete the last tissue level and ojas. The link to the endocrine system is extremely intimate. If the shukra is deficient, the hormone system will become imbalanced.

Therefore, the basic therapeutic approach is to strengthen and nourish the body. Hormone-supporting plants can be used to support the basic need to strengthen the whole body and the basic tissue level of shukra. Often, when this seventh level is affected, the tissue level of women, called the artava dhatu, is affected. Many times, shukra is given as seminal fluid in the man and artava as the egg and vaginal fluids in the woman. My teachers make this distinction: shukra is the reproductive tissues and fluids of both sexes and the artava dhatu is subservient to the shukra dhatu, yet stands apart and is not a "sub-dhatu." It is the tissue level that is related to the vagina and uterus and their tissues and excretions, not reproduction. Hence, the artava is involved in almost all gynecological problems. Shukra is involved with hormone and fertility problems. In this regard, shukra remains as the most subtle tissue level and artava is related and fed by the menstrual system, or srota. These are technical aspects, but interesting nonetheless.

It is also important to recognize that any problem in menstruation involves the plasma tissue level, because menstruation is a subtissue of the plasma dhatu, as is lactation. Any problem in menstrual fluid or in nursing indicates a deficiency in the plasma tissue level. Correcting the problem at its roots is more effective than treating the symptoms. Hence, the plasma dhatu should be looked at whenever there is a problem in menstruation.

Another primary point is that of vata being the primary dosha or humor. Vata has this distinction because the other two doshas cannot move or function without vata. The other name of vata is *vayu,* or "wind." *Vayu* is synonymous with prana, the life-force. Additionally, the *apana vayu* is always involved in the disease process—most especially in all reproductive and gynecological problems. Thus, one of the most effective treatments for women is to work directly on the vayu or prana srota. The prana srota (system) is called the *nadi* system in hatha yoga and is very much like the meridian system in Chinese medicine.

By working directly on the pranic channels of the body, vata can be moved and stimulated. This is one of the best treatment methods to achieve immediate relief from pain or discomforts. This method is called pranic healing and has existed in Ayurveda and yoga for many thousands of years. I have explained how to use this method by itself and with Ayurveda in two previous books.[1] Systems that work directly on the vata are Reiki, "hands-on healing," "universal energy," and others. Pranic healing, in the context of the yogic and Ayurvedic systems, has advantages over the other systems, which, in their most fundamental sense, are the same.

The primary advantage of using pranic healing is that it is a part of the whole science of yoga, of which Ayurveda is a part. In this use of the word, "yoga" refers to the Vedic tradition of reuniting the individual with the universal mind. Hatha yoga, which is actually related to Ayurveda as part of Ayurvedic lifestyles, is not the yoga to which I refer. The use of pranic healing according to a real medical system—one which intimately understands the science of prana

---

[1] Atreya, *Practical Ayurveda: Secrets of Physical, Sexual & Spiritual Health* (York Beach, ME: Samuel Weiser, 1998), and *Prana: The Secret of Yogic Healing* (York Beach, ME: Samuel Weiser, 1996).

and has never rejected it—has many advantages for those wishing to achieve precise results. For those wishing to use a general supportive system, Reiki and other systems usually give good results, depending on the practitioner's skill.

The main way Ayurveda uses the pranic currents is through the *marma* points. Marma therapy is a subbranch of Ayurvedic massage and is used to heal disease. In this way, a woman can heal doshic imbalances in the three humors directly, by balancing the vata through pranic currents. *Marma* means "hidden" or "secret," and provides a door to different channels. By stimulating a marma point, many gynecological problems can be relieved. This is very similar to the Chinese acupressure system. Yet, here again, it fits beautifully into a whole medical system—Ayurveda. I have explained in some detail how to work on the marmas and the systems and organs they balance in *The Secrets of Ayurvedic Massage*.[2]

Working on the subtle anatomy is a very effective way to balance the body and often provides the most immediate relief from discomfort. It is beyond the scope of this work to indicate every possibility in which the pranic currents can be used. However, books on pranic healing and marma therapy provide information for those interested in this effective way to harmonize the vata dosha directly.

Please consider every factor in your life before taking a therapeutic action. I picked up a recent book that purported to teach Ayurveda the other day, and was horrified to find that, after a lengthy explanation of everyone's uniqueness, a "cookbook" followed that gave all these "unique" people the same treatment! This is not Ayurveda. Understand the signs of your body; look at the wastes. Figure out which systems are involved. Learn about your body and the information that it is giving you. *All the information is there*! You must simply learn how to understand that information. Ayurveda provides this understanding.

---

[2] Atreya, *The Secrets of Ayurvedic Massage* (Twin Lakes, WI: Lotus Press, 1999).

CHAPTER FOUR

Imbalances and the Disease Process

What is known as the mind is, after all, always like a restless monkey.
Everybody knows that a restless mind is the channel of
endless troubles; whereas one is happy in sleep in the
absence of such restlessness.

—Tripura Rahasya

The classics of Ayurveda state that all diseases begin with the three humors. The disease process begins with a disturbance in one of the three humors, which may or may not lead to the aggravation of the other two humors. This disturbance or aggravation disrupts the metabolic function of the body. The humors can be disrupted from either physical or mental disturbances. Of the two, the mental has greater potential strength, according to Ayurveda.

The humoral point of view was also used in Europe until the Industrial Revolution, 200 years ago. Our own Western medicine has developed out of the humoral theory. It was the dominant medical explanation for thousands of years, beginning in India with Ayurveda, then spreading to Prussia, Greece, Italy, and the rest of Europe. While this point of view has been out of fashion for the last 200 years, it is once more becoming popular in the Western naturopathic circles, because it offers a more comprehensive view and treatment of an individual. Ayurveda, on the other hand, has never rejected the humoral theory and has practiced medicine according to it for over 5,000 years. Ayurveda also recognizes the validity of the biochemical model and is, consequently, the most comprehensive system available.

The ancient Ayurvedic texts state that, of the three humors, the *vata dosha* causes the majority of disease—about 70 percent of all illness. The *pitta dosha* causes about 20 percent and the *kapha dosha* causes about 10 percent. Therefore, the majority of preventative therapies in Ayurveda are orientated toward balancing the vata dosha.

Ayurveda explains that one or two of the humors will naturally be dominant in the natal constitution and that one (or one of the two) dominant humor(s) will tend to increase. It is natural for it to do so. Ayurveda tries to prevent this increase from happening. Preventing this increase is called "preventive medicine" in Ayurveda. If one or two of the humors increase, it is known as an "imbalance," or the beginning of the disease process.

The humors accumulate for a large variety of reasons—everything from stress in the workplace, to the wrong kind of meditation practice, to poor dietary habits. The main point of Ayurveda is to prevent them from becoming unbalanced (i.e., accumulating). This is why there is such an emphasis on lifestyle therapies and diet. It is what we do every day that creates health or disease by balancing or imbalancing the humors.

Second, if a humor does increase and begins to cause a disruption in the metabolism, we should treat it immediately to prevent it from disrupting the other two humors. As a humor increases, it begins to either overpower or overfeed another humor. When this happens, the treatment becomes more complicated. The more humors involved, the more difficult the treatment is going to be.

Normally, it is vata that is behind the disease process, because it is the principle of movement in the body and the mind. All external kinds of stress and movement aggravate the internal force of vata. Vata is irregular and unstable by nature, and is therefore easily disturbed.

Each of the humors is said to "live" primarily in one place in the body. This can be taken both metaphorically and literally, because the three humors permeate the entire body, yet the first signs of trouble or of increase occur in their "home" location. The vata humor lives in the large intestine (colon); the pitta humor lives in the small intestine (duodenum); and the kapha humor lives in the stomach.

The disease process has six stages. Ayurveda states that a humor will accumulate in its home, then become disturbed or aggravated. Next it fills it up or floods that home and moves out into the home of another humor, tissue level, or organ. Disease results, leading perhaps to a chronic problem or a complication that includes another disease. These are the six steps of the disease process:

1. Accumulation;
2. Disturbance;
3. Flood;
4. Movement;
5. Manifestation;
6. Complications.

For instance, vata may first collect in the colon and cause dryness (constipation, mild PMS), become disturbed (irregular PMS, irregular menses, constipation), fill the colon (strong PMS, cramping pain, irregularity, migraines), then move up either to the small intestine (pitta) or the lungs (kapha) or both (infections, discharges, pain, yeast imbalances, strong PMS). This then manifests as a disease in Western medicine (cysts, leukorrhea, PDI, chronic PMS, endometritis, etc.). This simply means that the symptoms have become so stable and acute as to be classifiable. Complications can result, thus, it is best to prevent all problems in the first or second stages.

Ayurveda recognizes three primary causes for the disturbance of the three humors and the beginning to the disease process. The first is our interaction with the environment through our senses. Our senses are the means by which we interact with the world and the people in it. This includes emotional factors and the abuse of the senses through over stimulation with mass media. It includes problems that arise from living in a modern city, like the overstimulation of sound, sight, smell, and, frequently, the lack of touch.

The second primary cause is called "failure of intelligence," which includes the wrong use of the body, the mind, and speech. These three factors include overeating, wrong eating habits, wrong living habits, incorrect use of the mind, and abusive habits of speech. In this context, "wrong" means inappropriate to your nature or constitution and has no direct moral implication. However, it is clearly understood that harming others, through words or deeds, is a "failure of intelligence" and as such, is destructive to health. Ayurvedic lifestyle therapies teach individuals how to live with intelligence, or in harmony with their unique natures.

The third factor is time. We can understand this as the process of aging and the diseases that arise from wear-and-tear on the body. This also includes the effects of seasonal changes on the body, something largely disregarded by modern practitioners. As a culture, we try to close ourselves off from, disassociate ourselves from, the seasons as much as possible. We insulate ourselves, with an attitude of fear and protectionism, from the changes of nature and we gravitate to the "perfect" climates around the globe that have as few seasonal changes as possible. Or we control the climates of our homes to create a "perfect" environment. Ayurveda clearly understands the role of the climatic changes in the disease process.

When any one of the three humors increases and starts to accumulate, it eventually floods or moves out of its home. Ayurveda recognizes three different pathways or routes through which the doshas (humors) move:

1. The *inner pathway,* or the digestive tract, beginning in the mouth and ending at the anus;
2. The *outer pathway,* which includes the superficial tissues (the skin) and the plasma and blood; and
3. The *middle pathway,* or the deep tissue level, including muscle, nerve, reproductive organs, and bone. It also includes immune-deficient problems.

This explanation makes it clear that chronic problems of menstruation are related to the second, or outer, pathway. The inner pathway is the easiest to cure, the outer the next easiest, and the middle the most difficult. Diseases must pass, however, from the first to third pathways, in order. Therefore, we have the possibility of stopping the disease process before it becomes serious. This is an important contribution from Ayurveda.

Ayurveda recognizes two different kinds of imbalances for any humor—toxic or nontoxic. This is explained below and indicates two different approaches in treatment. This differentiation is not clearly understood in Western herbalism and is frequently overlooked. Understanding this can significantly change the treatment approach.

Nontoxic Imbalances (Nirama):
This is the actual disease process, the accumulation of a humor that imbalances the metabolism, without any foreign matter (toxin) involved. This is the normal understanding in the biochemical approach to medicine, which seldom recognizes the accumulation of toxic matter. Ayurveda usually treats this kind of imbalance by first treating the natal humor and then the symptoms (or vikruti) of the person. This is often done simultaneously.

When the disease process is still free of toxic matter, it is much easier to eliminate or stop. Often, dietary changes alone are sufficient to stop a disease from beginning, if no toxins are present. Nontoxic states are generally clear and easy to diagnosis. They tend to be less complicated and more straightforward to treat.

Toxic Imbalances (Sama):
The toxic state of disease, or the presence of foreign matter in the disease process, is more common. In fact, it is so common that, in Ayurveda, most diseases are said to result from the presence of *ama,* or toxins, in the system. Toxins are simply undigested food that accumulates in the digestive tract and putrefies. In the act of rotting, it becomes toxic.

These toxins seldom remain in the digestive tract, however. They are usually absorbed into the blood stream and distributed freely throughout the body.

Once these toxins are in the body, they inhibit or impair the normal metabolic function, both on a cellular level and on a general metabolic level. This activity is the root cause of most chronic diseases, according to Ayurveda. These toxins can also lower the immune response, because the system must constantly fight the toxic presence in the body. Diseases with toxins are more difficult to treat and are often hard to diagnosis. Chemicals in food, water, and medication are generally considered to be toxins. In Ayurveda, the basic procedure is to first purify the body before undergoing long treatments—or at least to do both at once.

Discerning the Presence of Toxins:
The easiest way to see if your body is toxic is to look at your tongue. If the tongue is coated with a slight film, you have toxins. The color of the coating is indicative of the humor involved:

> Gray or brown indicates vata accumulation with the toxins;
> Yellow or green indicates pitta accumulation with the toxins;
> and White indicates kapha accumulation with the toxins.

Other signs of toxic accumulation in the body are bad breath, pimples, skin rashes, constipation, diarrhea, congestion, excess mucus, very smelly stools, smelly sweat, smelly or yellow urine, smelly vaginal discharges, chronic low energy, allergies of any kind, low immune response, frequent colds and fevers, low-grade fevers, and Chronic Fatigue Syndrome. All of these indicate various levels of toxins in the body. Before treating acute symptoms (such as cramps or a yeast infection), the level of toxins should be determined and addressed. It is also helpful to determine which disease pathway the toxins become lodged in the body.

Digestive problems—everything from constipation, to bloating, to food sensitivities—are indicative of the Inner Pathway. Blood, plasma, and skin problems are indicative of the Outer Pathway. This includes any kind of menstrual problem that is associated with the blood. It also relates to problems in the lymphatic system and water retention. Generally, problems in the vagina and uterus are related to this pathway, indicating that the cause may come from the Inner Pathway. Fibroids and cysts are common in the Outer Pathway, as are benign tumors.

Nerve, muscle, and bone-marrow problems are indicative of the Middle Pathway. This includes immune function and reproductive problems related to the ovaries. Cancer falls under this category, as does any rheumatic disease. Arthritis is also included. Many chronic menstrual problems tend to have migrated here over time.

It is also worthy to note that disease moves into the seven tissue levels, or dhatus. When a dosha (humor) moves into a dhatu level, it creates problems in that tissue level. Here again, the progress of disease is progressive through the tissues. Disease doesn't just jump to the seventh level of reproductive tissues. It must move through the other six levels. Recognizing the dhatu that is disturbed can help to identify the progress of the disease. *Dhatus are the sites of disease.* Generally menstrual problems are related to the blood level (rasa dhatu) and are not difficult to treat, if caught early. Fertility relates to the seventh level and requires long-term tonics and strengthening after toxins are removed.

CHAPTER FIVE

A Modern Look at the Hormone System

*She is light—One without a second;
and yet She appears divided to Her own creatures,
because of the veil of illusion.*

—Tripura Rahasya

Before proceeding further, it is helpful to understand the function of the endocrine system, commonly known as the hormone system. This information is significant because it affects the body on all levels and in all manners.

Men, in general, assume that only women have hormones. Men assume that they have only benign chemicals in their bodies. The word "hormone" surfaces frequently when a man is not interested in understanding a woman, or when he is having his own "period." When a man says, "It's hormonal," it generally implies only negative qualities and is a kind of "put down" that indicates a pseudo-superiority. It is rare today to find a woman who has not heard some negative comment about "hormones" from a man—or even, at times, from another woman.

Let's look at the social implications here before going into the actual physical functions of the body. There is only one reason why some people "put down" others, male or female—the lack of love and the desire to receive love. This is the bottom line. This is the root cause of fighting, of conflict, of emotional pain. If people feel well and are happy, they will not attack or make hurtful comments about others. The complexity of human relationships is beyond the scope of this book, yet they are important to your health. Hence, understand that, if a man or woman insults you or makes you feel badly, it is because they feel unloved and are unable to give love—they are in pain. Notice when you strike out at another how you feel. Are you feeling loved? Are you happy? These are fundamental questions that need to be addressed before anything else.

A man using the word "hormone" in a negative way implies a cultural enigma, or that he thereby gains a brief moment of feeling superior, or that he lives in an emotional wasteland. Men are trained to be callous and unfeeling in order to succeed in life. They block out and reject love, sentiments, feelings, and inner well-being. In order to do this, they have to cut themselves off from their own bodies (hormones) and feelings. They move slowly, as they grow older, into a deeper emotional wasteland and only experience brief moments of relief through material gains or sexual encounters.

As long as this social stereotype exists, we must understand that it is just that—a stereotype. Society, men and women, perpetuate the enigma of the insensitive, unfeeling male. And, unfortunately, many men actually conform to the stereotype.

Some insight into this problem can be gained by noticing how many women's problems can be linked to the male gender:

MENstruation
MENopause
MENtal breakdown
GUYnecology
HIMmorrhoids

This joke shows us that the best attitude to have is a light one! In essence, the roles of men and women are products of our society and cannot effectively be changed without a general raising of consciousness. As this is not about to happen soon, it is best to understand something about the body. Understand that chemical messengers—hormones—

are present in every function of the human body and are present in equal proportion in men and women. Men also have a monthly cycle and are prone to moods, irritability and depression. But, as they live in a male-dominated society in which these symptoms are unacceptable, they tend to blame other people or other things for the biochemical realities of their own bodies. (Living in an emotional wasteland is not supportive.)

What is a hormone—this enigmatic beast that is blamed by so many (male and female) for their troubles? What is this all-powerful force that can bring joy or sorrow so quickly? Well, actually, no one knows.

Oh, yes, doctors will often tell you otherwise. Yet, in the scientific community, there is great honesty about the actual lack of understanding of the endocrine function. Although much is known, much is still mysterious. It must be stressed that the hormonal function is multi-dimensional and cannot be reduced to "this does that." It is more appropriate to say, "this does that and that and that, which changes that and that and that, or so we think." This is precisely the attitude that research scientists have. It is also helpful to understand that the medical community is clearly divided into two levels—research and practitioners. Unfortunately, there is often a huge gulf between current research and common practice. The responsibility is ours to bridge them.

Here is what is known (in a purposefully simplified version). Endocrine glands are glands that secrete something directly into the blood stream. Exoctine glands secrete something through a duct, like the saliva or sweat. A few organs, like the pancreas, have both an endocrinel and exocrinel function. Endocrine glands secrete messengers, or *hormones*. These are often called *factors*, as they are the main factors, or links, for a metabolic function.

The endocrine system works very closely with the nervous system. As the nervous system is primarily related to the vata dosha—the humor of movement—much of the hormonal function relates to vata. As pitta is primarily related to metabolic change and control in the body, those endocrine glands and hormones which directly control metabolism relate to pitta. Examples will be given as we proceed.

So in essence, a hormone is a tiny messenger. When you eat an apple, a hormone is responsible for releasing the right kind of saliva, the right kind of stomach acids, and so on, throughout the whole digestive process. *Hormones are behind every function in your body.* The reproductive functions and menstruation of women are only one aspect of the hormonal system. Hence, anything that disturbs other aspects of the endocrine system *will tend to disrupt the menstrual cycle.* These include dietary, climatic, and emotional disruptions.

The first part of the endocrine system is actually not an endocrine gland, per se. It is the front part of the brain located on the floor of the third ventricle, the hypothalamus. It is connected to the thalamus and the pituitary gland and serves to bridge them. Thus it is one of the main connections between the nervous system (thalamus) and the hormonal system (pituitary). The hypothalamus controls body temperature, hunger, thirst, water balance, and sexual function, among other things. It is related to emotions and sleep, and governs all of this by regulating the automatic functioning of the nervous system through the pituitary gland. Not all of its functions are completely understood. Both vata and pitta help to control the hypothalamus.

The second part of the endocrine system is the pituitary gland (also called the hypophysis, just to confuse us). This is the brain of the hormonal system. It releases a complex variety of hormones that control growth, protein synthesis, sexual functions, and metabolic function in general. It actually controls so many hormone secretions that not all have been isolated or understood. It controls these secretions by receiving information from the brain (the hypothalamus either stimulates or inhibits) and the many other endocrine glands, via a complex feedback system. Both vata and pitta help to control the pituitary gland.

The third endocrine gland is the pineal gland. The role of the pineal gland is perhaps the one least understood by modern allopathic medicine. The pineal gland produces melatonin (along with serotonin). Melatonin has become popular in the mid-90s as a health supplement. In fact, there is much that is unknown about the function of these two hormones. They are known to interact with the adrenals, thyroid, testes, and ovaries. While theories abound, much more research needs to be done, since any hormonal imbalance can greatly affect the whole endocrine system. Ayurveda considers that one major function of the pineal gland is to link the physical and the subtle bodies. (The subtle body of yoga and Ayurveda includes the etheric, emotional, astral, and mental bodies). As such, large doses of melatonin could weaken or disturb this delicate balance, perhaps causing mental disorders. This may explain why many people (especially men) have vivid nightmares after taking melatonin. In Ayurveda, the vata sub-dosha, called prana vayu, directly controls this gland.

The fourth gland is the thyroid. It is related primarily to pitta, and controls the basic metabolic function of the body. It also controls growth in the young (a vata function) and has a role in regulating calcium in the blood. Not all of the functions of the thyroid are understood.

The fifth endocrine function is controlled by the parathyroids. They are related primarily to pitta and regulate the levels of calcium and phosphorus in the blood. This balance is critical for good bone growth and maintenance. Some aspects of the parathyroid glands are not completely known.

The sixth endocrine gland is the thymus. Much of its role remains a mystery to modern science. It is known to play a role in growth and immune function. Ayurveda considers the thymus to be related to kapha and, to some extent, to the concept of ojas. According to Ayurveda, the thymus continues to play an important role in adults. There is also a relation to the sub-vata, called vyana vayu, which controls balance in the body.

The adrenal glands are often given as the next endocrine glands. The functions of the adrenals are probably the least understood by laymen, yet they are the most important to overall health. Their simplified functions include the immune function, digestive metabolism, water metabolism, sexual metabolism, and nervous-system function. They also have a very important function as a transmitter throughout the body and functions as a feedback system to the pituitary gland. They are intimately related to the nervous system because of this feedback function. In Ayurveda, the function of the adrenal glands is primarily related to vata, then to kapha (through the kidneys and the water metabolism), and finally to pitta (through general metabolic balance). All three humors play a role in adrenal functioning, which should indicate their importance to us. During premenopause and in menopause, the adrenal glands completely take over the production of progesterones and are responsible for most estrogen production after menopause. They are thus very important for the health of women throughout their lives. One of the hormones produced in these glands is the now-famous DHEA. Because the function of the adrenal glands is so complex, some of their role in the body is not completely understood.

The eighth endocrine gland is the pancreas, which functions as both a ducted and ductless gland. It is related to kapha in its ducted function and to pitta in its hormonal function. The organ itself is given in Ayurveda texts as a kapha in nature, due to its relation to the water metabolism. The pancreas works closely with the adrenal gland to digest carbohydrates (complex sugars), protein, and fat. It is the adrenal gland that controls this function, but it is the pancreas that secrets the bile necessary to digest these nutrients (a pitta function).

Finally, we have the testes and ovaries. Both have a known relation to immunological function, supporting the Ayurvedic understanding that the seventh dhatu (tissue level) is the source of ojas, or immunity. Abuse weakens the immune system—not only overindulgence in intercourse, but sex without love and unnatural uses of the sex organs.

The function of the group of hormones known as estrogen are activated by the follicle-stimulating hormone (FSH) which is released from the pituitary gland. When FSH comes to the ovaries, estrogen production increases and an egg ripens and becomes ready to be released. The increase in estrogen prompts the uterine lining (endometrium) to thicken to receive the fertilized egg. The thickening of the uterus lining in turn activates the production of another hormone in the pituitary, the luteinizing hormone (LH). LH triggers the release of the now-ready egg (ovulation) and the production of the second main hormone, progesterone. The function of progesterone is to further prepare the uterine lining to receive the fertilized egg. If no egg is fertilized and implanted, the production of progesterone declines and the thickened uterine lining is shed in menstruation.

The ovaries produce not only estrogens and progesterone, but also several hormones necessary for the growth of a child in the womb. The ovaries also control lactation after birth. The inability to nurse can indicate an imbalance in ovarian function (the seventh tissue level). The ovaries work closely with the pituitary gland to regulate menstruation, fertility, pregnancy, and emotional harmony. The vata humor has the closest relation to the regularity of the cycle and timing of both menstruation and pregnancy (creation). Pitta is closest to the function of actual menstruation (transformation). Kapha is related to fertility, the ovum, and unity (love).

In addition to the main endocrine glands, there are other organs which produce hormones important to bodily functions. Each produces a significant hormone or hormonal group, of which a deficiency can result in illness, although this relationship may not be apparent. These are the gastrointestinal tract, the kidneys, the skin, and something called prostaglandins. Prostaglandins occur throughout the body in various tissues, organs, and fluids. They control many functions of the body. The organs to which they relate are kapha in nature (womb, lungs, brain, kidneys) and the fluids in the body are all of a kapha nature. The effect of taking estrogenic medications—birth control pills, ERT, or HRT—on the prostaglandins is not completely known and should be questioned carefully.

Table 3 gives a summary of endocrine function. To the best of my knowledge, this information is current. However, the field of hormone research is always changing. New hormones may have been identified or new functions may have been discovered for old ones. Table 3 reflects the current state of research at the time of my writing.

Table 3. Summary of Endocrine Functions and Relations

GLAND	HORMONE SECRETED	FUNCTIONS	DOSHA RELATION
Hypothalamus	Release factors for STH, TSH, FSH, LH, PRL, ACTH, MSH that are secreted from the pituitary; and secretes Vasopressin and Oxytocin to the pituitary	Stimulates the secretion and release of pituitary hormones; inhibits these same hormones from being secreted; Vasopressin and Oxytocin are made here	*Vata*: Prana Vayu, *Pitta*: Alochaka Pitta *Kapha*: Tarpaka Kapha is not directly related, yet it provides the cerebral fluid in which the brain functions
Pituitary	Somatotropin (STH), Thyrotropin (TSH), Follicle-Stimulating (FSH), Luteinizing (LH), Prolactin (PRL), Adrenocorticotropin (ACTH), Melancyte Stimulating (MSH), Vasopressin (ADH), Oxytocin	Releases all the hormones given on the left to regulate metabolism, growth, protein synthesis, the thyroid gland, controls ovaries and testes, estrogen and progesterone, lactation, adrenal function, blood pressure, kidney function	Same as above.

Table 3. Summary of Endocrine Functions and Relations (cont.)

Pineal	Melatonin (MLT), Serotonin	Influences cyclic activities in metabolism and sexual maturity; functions are not completely understood	*Vata*: Prana Vayu
Thyroid	Thyroxine, Calcitonin	Regulates basal metabolism, growth, and development	*Vata*: Udana Vayu, Pitta in general is related to the thyroid, but especially Pachaka and Sadaka Pitta
Parathyroid	Parathyroid Hormone	Regulates the level of calcium & phosphorus in the blood	*Vata*: Udana and Vayu *Pitta*: Ranjaka Pitta
Thymus	Thymosin, Thymopoietin, and others	Influences the lymphatic glands, general immunity, cell immunity, through production of T-cells and growth; functions are not completely understood	*Vata*: Prana Vayu, Vyana Vayu *Kapha*: Avalambaka Kapha
Adrenal	Glucocorticoids (DHEA and others), Mineralocorticoids, estrogens, progesterone, androgens	Influences carbohydrate, protein, and fat metabolism; anti-inflammatory and immunosupressive; regulates sodium, potassium, and water metabolism in general; supplements the action of the ovaries and testes	*Vata*: Samana Vayu, Apana Vayu *Pitta*: Pachaka Pitta *Kapha*: Keldaka Kapha

Table 3. Summary of Endocrine Functions and Relations (cont.)

Pancreas	Insulin, Glucagon	Helps utilize glucose, regulates blood sugar through the secretion of these two hormones, which are opposite in action	*Vata*: Samana Vayu *Pitta*: Pachaka Pitta *Kapha*: Kledaka Kapha
Ovaries	Estrogen, Progesterone, Relxin	Regulates the development of female sexual organs, fertility, controls menstruation with FSH and LH, relaxes pelvic muscles and ligaments	*Vata*: Apana Vayu *Pitta*: Ranjaka Pitta

It should be stressed that, while modern science has made huge progress in understanding the individual functions of the endocrine glands and hormonal secretions, much less progress has been made toward an understanding of the complex interrelationships between these glands. In fact, the overall functioning of the body is so dependent on these hormones that even a vitamin or mineral deficiency can play havoc with the body, because an endocrine gland may be affected by this deficiency. Problems of the thyroid are a clear example.

In this aspect, Ayurveda can provide us a much better overview of the total functioning of the endocrine system. This is not to discount the biochemical understanding of allopathic medicine, but rather to provide a broader context in which to use the biochemical information. Used in conjunction with an overview, such information can increase our health. Used within the confines of a purely mechanical model, this information can produce huge imbalances and dependencies in the body. This is exactly what happened to my own mother.

Women should be aware that taking any chemical or "natural" hormone can have many unknown effects on the body. Some of these effects are known, but many are not. The modern medical community uses percentages and averages to justify the use of these hormone medications, knowing full well that emotional imbalance, water retention, and cancer of the breast and uterus can become more likely. They justify these risks by citing the supposed "benefits."

What is now held as common practice, however, certainly will change in a decade or two, as it has always done in allopathic medicine. Women should question if they want to be guinea pigs for future generations. Other options are available that are generally scoffed at or suppressed for very specific reasons—arrogance or greed. In fact, over 90 percent of the research being conducted today is paid for by large pharmaceutical companies. Many lives have been saved because of this research, but many lives have been destroyed. It is difficult to know into which category you will fall. The primary point here is that data and facts collected by the United States government show that herbal medicine is several thousand times safer than current pharmaceutical treatments (see Introduction).

While it is true that not all the effects of plants—primary or secondary—are known, with proper administration, they at least are not life-threatening or damaging. The human body is able to process and eliminate organic plant compounds, which is not the case with manufactured medications. It is also true that these plant compounds are often limited in their ability to correct major problems, primarily because treatment is not begun soon enough.

It should also be pointed out that the hormone group of estrogen and progesterone do not exist in a natural state outside of the human body, either in animals or in plants (although some companies would like you to believe they do). The advantage to plants is that many herbs provide a simple steroid base that is the base of all hormones in humans and animals. The use of "hormone-promoting" herbs provides just that—support for hormone production. The disadvantage is that, in some cases, these compounds may not be strong enough to make a direct change in a seriously imbalanced system. The advantage is that they are not strong and invasive. They work to support the body's natural functions and so aid the body to balance itself. This brings a better state of health, in the opinion of Ayurveda, because no outside person or agency can know which of the many hundreds of hormones to produce and administer, or in what quantity. In most cases, plant steroids provide an increase of raw materials in your body, so that it can do the work on its own.

The workings of the body are so complex that, as a totality it is not completely understood. We have not been able to "create" a human being yet—although the possibility is coming closer. This should cause us to question the horrifying possibilities, considering who is paying for this research and what their motivation may be. At the foundation of this complex physical/mental/emotional functioning is the tiny hormone. Playing around with your hormones may give some noted benefits, yet it is far more likely to reduce your quality of life faster than almost any other treatment used today.

Strangely enough, it is the quality of life that has been used to promote hormone replacement therapy since the mid-60s. Several studies note that *60 percent of women in the United States stop taking hormones by the third month* due to the uncomfortable side effects. This should cause us to question why so many women do not want to have the quality of their lives improved.

In most traditional cultures—indeed in our own until the Industrial Revolution—menopause happened relatively effortlessly for the majority of women. A small percentage had difficulties. Even today, as many as half of all women have little problem with declining hormone production. On the contrary, many women are elated and happy about the change. These facts and attitudes, however, do not create an industry, and are therefore ignored.

CHAPTER SIX

How Substances Work in the Body

---

*Her Majesty, the Absolute, remains always aware of Her perfection
and oneness. Though Herself immutable, She appears mutable to
Her own creatures just as a magician beguiles the audience
with his tricks, but remains himself undeceived.*

—Tripura Rahasya

In order to understand the therapeutic approach of Ayurveda, we must understand something of the effects of plants and foods on the body, as this forms the basis for all treatment.

In theory, the substances that we ingest are supposed to nourish us—at least, this is the general concept that most people have. In reality, this is usually not the case. Ordinarily, we only absorb and utilize a percentage of what we ingest. This percentage varies greatly according to many factors and is often indicative of our general overall health.

Hence, the fundamental approach of Ayurveda revolves around the *capacity* of our digestion, before it concerns itself with what is being ingested. This concept is often foreign to modern medical practitioners, but its logic is undeniably sound. Of what good is something if our body lacks the ability to digest it and assimilate it? This is true for herbal medicines, as well as for foods.

The capacity to digest a substance involves a wide array of systems in the body. The digestive process includes the nervous system, the hormone system, blood circulation, proper respiration for the oxidation of blood and tissues, lubrication provided by the water metabolism, and so on. In fact, every system of the body is involved to some degree in the digestive process. This is one reason why Ayurveda stresses the health of the digestive process so heavily. The other reason is that the digestive system is the home of each of the three humors, those forces that cause disease in the body.

It is pure ignorance, no matter which medical system you use, to think that digestion is isolated to the digestive tract and organs alone. No medical system advocates this point of view, but it is only Ayurveda that places the correct importance on it. Ayurveda also understands the interrelationship of all the different systems of the body and the process that food has on developing the mind, the emotions, and the physical aspects of the body.

The basic building block of the physical body is food, or the substances that we ingest regularly. If poor-quality food is ingested, our health can only end up being poor. However, even if a person eats well, they may not be able to assimilate the food due to the complicated relationship of the digestive system to the other systems of the body. The foremost system in creating digestive problems is the nervous system.

Here again, it is vata that controls the nervous system. Probably the greatest disturbance, after the actual quality of our food, is the state of the nervous system in the body. People often mistake the lack of visible stress as health. However, repressed feelings and unresolved emotions can be stored in the nervous tissue and disrupt the function of vata in the body. This can greatly diminish the power of assimilation. Generally, the disturbance of vata will appear in the digestive system, as mental agitation, or as a disruption in the endocrine system. In all of these cases, a woman can experience problems in her cycle.

With this in mind, we can now actually look at how the two different systems, modern and ancient, treat how the body processes different substances.

The Biochemical View

Allopathic medicine is often called mechanical medicine. This represents a view that the sum of the parts make a whole. The relation of the parts to the whole and the function of the whole as a whole is seldom, if ever, acknowledged. With this view, the scientist tries to understand the whole by learning about its parts. The idea is that, if you understand the parts, you will understand the whole.

When presented in this simplistic manner, the approach seems absurd to many. Nevertheless, there is solid ground for this view and much good has come from its use. As I mentioned before, this view is respected in Ayurveda as a *partial* view.

The partial nature of this view becomes apparent when we look at the effects of synthetic medications on the body. By synthetic medications, I mean substances manufactured in a laboratory, whether or not they are made from organic substances. Their chemical structure may be identical, nevertheless they are dead, inert substances. These inert substances were developed for a reason.

Throughout history, plants have been used as medicine. Yet the therapeutic potency and reliability of the plants varied greatly with the season and method of growing and harvesting. When the Industrial Revolution began in the late 18th century, one of the prime goals was to find a way to stabilize the source of medicines so that more accurate and reliable results could be achieved. An admirable task for humanity. Similarly, the storage of medicines had always been a problem. And so, over the years, methods were developed in which the therapeutic substances of plants could be extracted and stored safely.

This approach reflects the mechanical view—that by understanding the active chemical or chemicals in a plant, one could understand the effect of the plant on disease and reproduce it. This logic is still followed today, even after decades of problems and side effects. At first, many major breakthroughs were made in the treatment of disease. And there are still breakthroughs being made today, but at what cost?

Many diseases were eradicated from society and many more have taken their place. Many senseless operations are performed daily across the country—everything from hysterectomies to the removal of tonsils. The body is treated as if it produced undesirable organs that could act as the source of disease. We are brainwashed into believing that modern medicine has eliminated the major causes of disease from the developed countries of the world.

This information is questionable. At best, we have substituted one set of diseases for another. The increase of various cancers, heart attacks, and hardening of the arteries alone is enormous. Yet, perhaps the most unpublicized and frightening fact is that the major cause of death worldwide is still viral infections—the flu. People are now becoming aware that viruses are becoming more and more resistant to antibiotics due to their blatant overuse by the medical community. One wonders why it takes six years of study and several years of internship to prepare doctors to prescribe the same antibiotic to a variety of people with a variety of problems.

We are now seeing a whole string of environmental diseases that result from the massive amounts of industrial pollutants in our food chain. Just one example of this: fifty-one of the thousands of chemicals used daily directly affect the endocrine system.[1] Most of these are what are called "estrogenic chemicals." They occur in pesticides, fertilizers, plastics, detergents, household cleaning products, canned foods, and even contraceptive creams. They are in PCBs (polychlorinated biphenyls). These chemicals now occur throughout the environment. They directly impair or overstimulate estrogen production, which is shown consistently in studies to promote cancers, tumors, and other growths in

---

[1] Theo Colburn, et. al., *Our Stolen Future* (New York: Penguin, 1997).

the body. Excess estrogen can cause anxiety and promote excessive fat synthesis (weight gain).

As pesticides and fertilizers have now penetrated every level of the food chain, both men and women are more and more prone to problems of the endocrine system—which we have seen controls the whole body. The rise of cancers can be correlated directly to foods and diets. Science knows this, but the information is kept out of the public media by people and companies that profit from the foods and products being sold. It should be noted that we are dependent on these same products in our daily life. What researchers know and what is made public is often very different. The books of John Robbins[2] present interesting information along these lines, especially about diet and nutrition.

With this information, it is hard to accept the rationale that science has truly eliminated disease from the planet. Wouldn't it be more accurate to state that science has replaced one set of diseases with another? Dr. Subhuti Dharmananda, a research scientist and the head of the Institute for Traditional Medicine and Preventive Health Care, had this to say in 1980 about the history of medicine:

> Where practiced, improved sanitation and proper diet have done more for health than any **medicine that has ever been used**. Few people seem to manage these conditions in their lives, and so medicines are required to perform a monumental task.[3]

Modern pharmaceuticals have been created to combat the problems of human society, most of which come from pollutants and bad habits. The leading cause of death today in India is dysentery, a viral infection caused by unsanitary conditions. In the United States, we have other kinds of pollutants that cause breast cancer, high blood pressure, and

---

[2] John Robbins, *Diet for a New World* (New York: Avon Books, 1992) and *Diet for a New America* (Walpole, NH: Stillpoint Publishing, 1987).

[3] Michael Tierra, *The Way of Herbs* (New York: Pocket Books, 1998) p. x.

other diseases. It is because of these external factors and poor eating habits that people generally fall ill. Heart disease is the leading killer of women over 50, yet the fact that diet and exercise have been clearly linked to heart disease does not prevent doctors from trying to treat the *result* of poor lifestyles. Hence, modern pharmaceuticals are designed to combat the *symptoms* of these diseases and not the causal factors of lifestyle or environment.

Here, then, is the major shift away from Ayurvedic philosophy: focusing on the symptoms, rather than on the origin of the symptoms. Science feels that, by finding the pathogen responsible for a symptom and eliminating it, they can restore health. This approach is limited to acute conditions. Daily observation shows again and again that the same symptoms recur after a treatment with synthetic drugs has effectively eradicated the pathogen from the body. Why then does the disease recur? Perhaps the true cause of the disease is not limited to a pathogen.

Let's look at a simplified version of how synthetic pharmaceutical products work in the body. These products are made to achieve quick, standard, consistent results. This means something that can be measured in one way or another, over and over again. If a substance can be manufactured or isolated to do this, then it becomes of value to science. These products have to be separated and isolated from other substances in order to measure them effectively. It also allows science to observe the effects of the isolated substance.

Through this process, the substance is rendered inert, dead. It is rendered inorganic (i.e., no longer occurring in its original state, as in nature). Its chemical structure remains the same, or extremely close, but it is considered dead by the human body. This can best be defined by its action in the body. These isolated synthetic substances have an invasive action in the body. They do not work with the body, but rather in spite of it. This is why these products have achieved miraculous effects against disease.

This, however, always has a price. This invasiveness—or breaking-and-entering—action always creates side effects. These secondary effects can be known or unknown. Modern science mainly uses one criteria for determining if a substance is safe or not: Is it carcinogenic? The question of whether a substance causes cancer is thus the primary factor in determining if that substance is safe for the treatment of disease. The other side effects are often not measured or investigated due to a lack of time and money. In fact, to know all the side effects of any given isolated substance, one would have to test each system, organ, and gland, and their functions in the body. And you would still never know how the total organic whole would respond to the isolated substance. (Note: There are other tests used as well, e.g., effects on the liver, etc. The above is a simplified version of pharmaceutical testing and is not meant to be critical, but rather to show the impossible task science faces in trying to know all of the effects on the body of an isolated substance.)

These substances do not have an innate intelligence that tells them which things belong in the body and which do not. They flood the cells (which cells depends on the medication being used) and enter forcibly to do their job. Another major test of scientific medicine is to see if the body can eventually eliminate most of the substance. If not, it is called toxic and considered to be a poison. The body is then faced with the task of rejecting the product and the pathogens it destroyed, a task the body is often unable to perform completely. Some small percentage of the medication remains in deep tissues or the organs of filtration.

Vitamin C can serve as a valuable example here. Vitamin C is known to be safe and beneficial when used correctly. In this example, we will use a synthetic vitamin C, which is the most common form of the vitamin in the United States. The synthetic vitamin must first confront the digestive tract in order to be dissolved and reduced to a usable form that can be absorbed into the plasma via the blood to nourish the cells. After all, everything happens in the cells.

But does your body have the enzymes necessary to break down and digest this man-made vitamin? Certainly a portion is able to be used, because laboratories have been able to observe the effects. So why is your urine always so yellow when you take vitamins? Because you are either unable to use, or do not need, this portion of the vitamin. Many people find it illogical to think that humans have the inherent enzymes to digest the many synthetic products that appear each year in our food chain. This is definitely worth considering, especially for those who have food allergies or sensitivities.

When the vitamin (or a percentage of it) is broken down and absorbed into the blood, it eventually reaches the cell, the core metabolic building block of the body. The cell has a wall made up of lipids and proteins that control the absorption of nutrients into the cell. Within the cell wall, there is a jellylike fluid called the cytoplasm. Within this fluid, hundreds of activities take place, according to the function of the cell and its location in the body. In this process, the cell wall or membrane plays a critical role. It allows certain things in and keeps other things out. It allocates certain openings to certain nutrients. This means that vitamin C has special openings and that, when you eat an orange, the vitamin C zooms through the plasma until it finds a cell opening for vitamin C that is free. It then enters and aids the metabolic process of the body.

Unfortunately, the synthetic vitamin C that we are using doesn't have a clue about these rules and it just pushes its way into the cell wherever it can find an opening. Being man-made, it has not received the instructions from Mother Nature but is either ignorant or inert. This is what natural medicine calls a dead substance, because it does not know how to function with the body; it does not know its natural role. It lacks intelligence. It lacks life. Intelligence and life are two principles that occur together throughout nature. They are called purusha and prakruti in Ayurveda.

When the vitamin C floods the cells—as in a high dose to fight a cold, or because you think it is good for health—the openings for other vitamins, minerals, and nutrients become blocked. This prevents the other nutrients from being absorbed for as long as the cell wall is flooded with vitamin C. Obviously, this is not an optimal situation. Fortunately, the body processes this vitamin C rather quickly and the openings are cleared for the other nutrients to come in—that is, unless you continue to take high doses.

Nonetheless, there is still the actual process of utilization within the cell. Many times, the cell cannot use or remove all of the product ingested. Fortunately, vitamin C seems to be almost completely used or rejected by the cell. If it is not, the basic metabolic function of the body is impaired and its ability to process simple things like cholesterol and carbohydrates is affected.

Studies have consistently shown that large, regular intakes of any vitamin actually cause a deficiency of that vitamin. Why? Because the body is continually flooded with it and looses the ability to produce it or utilize it from natural foods. This also leads to other problems.

What if we were to substitute the birth control pill for vitamin C? What might be the effect? Or an estrogenic substance? The target of these synthetic pills is the endocrine system and the cells that live there. Is your body able to effectively use or eliminate this pill year after year? What effect will this drug have on the cell membranes? What other hormones or nutrients is this medication preventing from entering the cell? These are legitimate questions for every woman to ask herself with respect to all synthetic products—everything from aspirin to antidepressants.

This effect is common knowledge and well known. The medical community justifies this by saying that the benefits are, on the whole, much greater than any negative effects. If you like to play the odds, then this argument may be acceptable. I do not consider myself to be a part of an average or a percentage. Consequently, I do not accept this kind of argument, provided that other alternatives are available for my health.

Another important factor is how modern scientific studies are performed and how they calculate their odds. There are three major biases that influence the results of any clinical study. These are called *selection biases*.

Here is an example of how this works. Consider a hypothetical study that shows that women who take estrogen (ERT) therapy have about 40 percent fewer heart attacks than those who don't. This sounds good, until you look at the selection biases. First, there is a *health bias*. Only women who are healthy, those with no history of heart, artery, or blood-pressure problems are allowed to participate in the study. This means the study is done with a group of people statistically low in heart-disease susceptibility—in other words, healthy women who are not likely to have heart attacks.

In addition, the women who participate in the study are statistically a different group of women than the national average that is used to determine that heart disease is the leading killer of women over a certain age. These women tend to be seeking good health. They eat better, exercise more often, go to the doctor more frequently. They have higher incomes and less stress than the national average. These are the most important factors in the prevention of heart disease. This can be called the *life-style bias*. Women are chosen who are living a supportive life that already prevents heart disease.

The third factor is called the *compliance bias* of the scientific community. This means that people who willingly participate in studies statistically benefit much more than those who are unwilling or not told that they are participating in a study. For example, compliant women given a placebo and those given an estrogenic medication both had 40 percent fewer heart problems, which indicates that the taking of *any* medication would result in a 40 percent reduction in heart disease.

It should be pointed out that all estrogenic compounds are contraindicated for women with any kind of heart or circulatory problem. The FDA has not approved any estrogenic medication for the treatment of heart disease. This makes one wonder why such a study—one that shows ERT to prevent heart attacks—was published in the media in the first place. Certainly it gives the false idea to women that estrogen prevents heart attacks, when there is a long clinical history that shows estrogen to be a major factor in causing heart problems of all kinds—a conclusion exactly the contrary to that produced by the media.

This is the state of affairs today. You should be aware that the continuing use of synthetic substances imbalances the vata dosha. They slowly impair the metabolic function, which imbalances the pitta dosha. In time, this results in the derangement of the kapha dosha. The regular consumption of synthetic products, either in the diet or as medication, is one of the major factors in the derangement of vata and so can be seen as a major cause of disease in modern society, according to Ayurveda. In Ayurveda, there is a special branch of medicine, called *Agadatantra,* which deals only with toxicology—the science of healing the body from poisons. Perhaps we can learn much from this branch today.

The Ayurvedic View

The Ayurvedic system cannot separate nutritional intake, the mental state, daily habits, your environment, and your deeper motivations in life from the medicine it prescribes. Ayurveda views the whole as inclusive of the parts, not as the sum of the parts. To understand the parts, one must understand the whole. The part reflects the whole and the whole is contained in the part. Hence, treatments evolve around the person and look to the parts as reflecting discord in the whole. Even when a disease's origins are not clear, a person can be treated "constitutionally," according to their natal nature. Anything that deviates from that nature is indicative of imbalance.

If you find a practitioner or book advocating treatment of the symptoms and not the constitution, be forewarned that it is not Ayurveda, but an aberration of the mother system. Ayurveda is often called the mother of all medicines, because it treats you like a loving mother, taking care of you on all levels. It is also called that because all medical systems have either been derived from it or taken knowledge from it, including modern medicine. It is a system so vast that it is hard to comprehend. Yet today many practitioners are using the name of Ayurveda and still practicing in a mechanical manner.

Plants have been used medicinally for as long as human beings have existed. Are they safe? Do they actually work? Medicinal plants are safe if used correctly and unsafe if used inappropriately. Plants work very well to heal basic imbalances of the metabolism and body, but are less effective in treating acute diseases that derive from poor living habits and ignorance (i.e., waiting too long to treat metabolic disorders in the body).

It is unrealistic to think that herbal medicine can be effective if you do not have a lifestyle and diet that support it. This is probably the main reason why modern medical science has been so unsuccessful in using traditional natural remedies in the traditional manner—because the whole environment must be supportive to the herbal treatment. This is why medical doctors who have embraced a "holistic" approach in the treatment of heart disease, obesity, and other diseases have such astounding results.

If you are not willing to take the responsibility, and the power that comes with that responsibility, into your own hands, then it is better to remain a percentage. Herbal treatments will seldom work if you are not willing to create a supportive environment in which they can function. It is the failure of each of us to be responsible that has led to the general dissatisfaction with medical practitioners today. While the medical industry as a whole has helped in this and played an important role, the responsibility of our own health lies in our hands. We have consistently chosen to give that power away to someone else who "knows better."

No one person knows more about your own body than you do. The more you listen, the more you will know. The failure to listen to your body will, sooner or later, cause disease and result in your losing control. This is common knowledge. Ask any woman who has suffered through a major operation because she said "yes" out of fear and ignorance. Operations are the most invasive thing you can have done to your body. This is not to say that surgery has not saved many lives. It saved my arm, which I can use today. Without surgery I would have only one arm.

Ayurveda provides a total context of living that supports herbal medicine. If you test the traditional formulas outside of the system you may not get very good results. However, it is very unlikely—no, *highly improbable*—that a medical system would continue to exist for over 5,000 years *if it didn't work.*

If you are tired of being treated as a percentage by modern forms of medicine, whether they are mechanical or natural, use Ayurveda. It has taken me years to really understand that everything is Ayurveda. Nothing is good or bad. All of life is included in the Ayurvedic understanding. *Ayurveda is the science of understanding the nature of things.*

When the whole system of Ayurveda is used, fantastic results can be achieved. The system addresses daily habits, nutrition, mental happiness, relations, career, the spirit, and finally, if needed, medicine. Ayurveda views medicine as a last resort, to be used when something has been wrong for some time and left unattended or been ignored. This is, in fact, the case with most of us. When I get sick, it is because I have ignored the signs that indicate a problem is on the way.

Another major problem, stemming from the Industrial Revolution, is that we have been encouraged to lose connection with our bodies. This is more the outcome of a purely material vision than a conscious effort by any segment of society. As a society, we have lost touch with our bodies and the knowledge of how to maintain them on a daily basis. This has become more critical over the last hundred years, as the migration to the cities accompanied the loss of traditional wisdom. Ayurveda has maintained this knowledge.

So what is the therapeutic approach of Ayurveda when we are confronted with a reoccurring or stable symptom, which we call a disease? Ayurveda uses a wide variety of plants and mineral substances to rebalance the total organism. The symptom is a secondary consideration from the Ayurvedic point of view. The symptoms or pathogens could not have taken root in the body if there had not been a deeper imbalance that provided the right environment. Hence, Ayurveda is always concerned with the root of disease. It perceives the root of all disease as an imbalance in the three humors or doshas. Treatment is structured around your natal constitution and any imbalance that may be "covering" that constitution.

In the West, we either do not have access to the mineral preparations that are traditionally used in Ayurveda, or they are considered "toxic" by modern medicine. This view causes one to question the methods, motivations, and financing of such studies that show these products to be "unsafe," when they have been used for thousands of years and are still used safely today in other parts of the world. In any case, although these mineral preparations are safe, they are also unavailable.

We are thus left with the plant kingdom and some modern preparations of minerals. The only mineral preparations that are easily assimilated by the body are those produced by the homeopathic system. These preparations tend to keep the original ingredient intact and yet render it in a form that can be used effectively by the body. I use these preparations in my practice frequently.

The plant kingdom can and does provide us with many medicines that help us balance and maintain health. The question then arises of why, if plants and medicinal herbs are so effective, do modern scientific studies often show their effect as limited or insubstantial? Why are these substances often inconsistent in their effect? And most importantly, what are the secondary effects? We know by now that it is virtually impossible for science to know of the multidimensional effects of any substance taken into the body (like a candy bar that is composed of synthetic products) because of the many chemicals present and because of the complexity of the metabolism. Why then are plant medications safer than synthetic medicines?

The answer to the first question I have already addressed. Plant medications need to be used in a supportive environment, both physically and mentally. They also work most effectively on a deeper level of the body to balance metabolic function rather than acute symptoms (although, when used correctly, they can be as effective in the treatment of acute symptoms).

The second question relates to modern procedures of testing and the usual practice of using an extract of the plant rather than the whole plant, so as to have a measurable quantity to study. This is very limiting, because a plant or herb can have twenty different "active ingredients" and hundreds of "inert" ingredients. The interaction of these different substances within any given plant is not really known, nor is the effect of the totality on any other organism, simply because there is no way to measure it. It is too complex. Unfortunately, very few clinical studies have taken place using the whole plant or a mixture of plants (outside of India and China). Therefore, we are left with traditional uses of plants as our therapeutic guide. Modern medicine is basically extracting an ingredient and comparing it to the traditional use of the plant, which will, of course, give vastly different results. In general, herbalists tend not to be able to finance billion-dollar studies, so this trend is not likely to end soon.

As to the question of secondary effects, there are many, and yet they tend to be supportive rather than destructive.

For example, an herb may have an effect of purifying the blood of toxins (oxygenating it), yet it may also have the secondary effect of promoting liver function and increasing the synthesis of vitamin B_{12}. The real problem in using herbs is that they are so well balanced and have so many effects that their usage can also be too broad.

The bottom line here is: Can your body effectively process herbal medicines? The answer is emphatically—yes! Plants do not impair digestion (when used correctly), nor do they assault your metabolic function in an invasive way. This discussion is, of course, limited to the use of medicinal plants and not narcotics like opium, marijuana, and others. This is not to say that these plants do not have value, but they are not the focus of this discussion and fall under a strictly medical application by a highly trained medical herbalist.

It is worthy to note that hormones do not exist in plants. There are phyto- (meaning "plant") steroids that form the basis for the production of many human hormones. They often act like hormones in the body. There are at least fifty-seven known phytosteroids. They are found in foods and in herbs. Their main sources are in oils, whole grains, nuts, and seeds. It is interesting to note that Ayurveda has a long history of using sesame oil to control vata and nourish the body. It is especially used in cases of weakness and rejuvenation.

We are given, by Mother Nature, medicines that not only support our metabolic function, but also work to correct it when needed. These substances are easily eliminated from the body if unused or unwanted. They do not create deficiencies of other nutrients in the body. Only if abused will they disrupt the nervous and endocrine systems. They are "whole medicines" offering not only specific chemicals, but also nutritional support through a wide variety of vitamins and minerals—something many of us now have to supplement in our diets because we do not take in foods and herbs in a natural state. Herbs offer a wide spectrum of ingredients, both active and inactive, that are supported by a natural balance of minerals and vitamins which help the ingredients to be absorbed and used by the body.

Ayurveda overcomes the problem of the varied use and actions of herbs by mixing them together into formulas. Through this method, practitioners can more effectively target a specific therapeutic reaction. They can also address lesser or secondary problems that may be contributing to the imbalance or disease. It is also possible to actually increase the digestive power and assimilation at the same time, which results in a better therapeutic action and increased nutritional support.

By using the traditional formulation methods, one can address a broad array of problems and correct many health problems. One can also target the root cause of disease, which may appear vague and insubstantial to the modern doctor because it addresses the metabolism or immunity, rather than organ function or pathogens. In essence, the correct use of an herbal formula is clinically impossible to measure and monitor by modern scientific means. Yet it can provide a comprehensive treatment for a living human being.

PART TWO

Ayurvedic Treatments

CHAPTER SEVEN

The Ayurvedic Method

*It is not an object to be perceived, nor described; how shall I
then tell you of it? You know the Mother only if you know the Self.*

—Tripura Rahasya

This section is *not* for the treatment of dangerous, life-threatening diseases. It is *not* for the treatment of undiagnosed illnesses. If you do not know what is the matter with your body, seek professional help first to determine the problem, then study your options. Some gynecological problems can have serious consequences on your long-term health. A book is no replacement for a living practitioner. However, a book can help you explore options once you know what you are up against—that is the purpose of this section—not to diagnose, but to offer my experience in treating certain types of problems using the Ayurvedic system.

It must be clearly understood that the approach presented here is oriented primarily toward balancing the constitution and metabolism. The effect of this is long-term health and the elimination of a variety of symptoms. While diseases are given according to category, the treatments are given not to address the symptoms, but to correct the metabolic imbalance that generally underlies the disease.

With such a general approach, the effectiveness of the formulas is questionable. My clinical experience shows that, by using these basic constitution-specific formulas, you come to expect a 70 to 80 percent success rate. In my own practice, I achieve a higher success rate because I can adjust the basic formulas to fit the individual more precisely.

Before starting the section on treatments, a word or two is needed about the Ayurvedic use of herbs and about my own experience with them. The Ayurvedic medical system uses a wide variety of medicinal preparations. Traditional methods change according to the constitution, the disease type, the location of the disease, the strength of the disease, and the person (age, mental state, and strength). When all these factors have been considered, a method of preparation and administration can be chosen. Ayurveda uses the juice, aerial parts, and roots of plants, depending on the treatment and the above-mentioned factors.

In this book, I have presented only one basic approach to using plants, one which is primarily effective for correcting chronic imbalances in the digestive, nervous, and endocrine systems—the general metabolic function of the body. I concentrate on the use of powdered plants, roots, fruits, seeds, and occasionally the flowers. I have done this for several reasons. Most of my clients come to me with chronic problems that they have either tried to treat in other ways or ignored until they were affecting their constitution. The availability of fresh plants and the ability to mix different parts of the plants, which is not possible in other forms of preparation were also factors. It is also stronger therapeutically to actually ingest the whole powdered plant than it is to brew a tea or make an extract of it.

Because of the elements peculiar to each kind of preparation, tinctures are best used to correct acute problems that need immediate attention, teas are best used for health maintenance, and powders are best used to nourish or to change deep, chronic problems. Tinctures are fast acting, because as they are composed primarily of ether and air (vata). They are quick to act, yet over the long term tend to imbalance vata. The advantage of tinctures is that they stay fresh for a long time and keep well when stored. In the process of making them, however, some of the inert or active principles of the plant may not be extracted. They are generally easy to use, to mix, and to gauge in dosage, and so are popular with many herbalists.

Teas, either infusions (steeping leaves or flowers in boiled water for twenty minutes) or decoctions (boiling roots or barks in water until the liquid is reduced to half) are mild and do not extract all the active principles of the plants. Some of the inert or active components of the plants may not be extracted. Teas are time-consuming to make and may be less effective if they are not fresh, or if they contain an insufficient amount of the plant being used for the therapy. Teas generally relate to the water and fire elements (water can hold both air and ether as well), depending on the plants used. Doses are harder to regulate because the amount of the plant used to make the tea is seldom weighed and so is subjective.

Tablets are another option. These are better from my point of view because, hopefully, they contain the part of the plant that has medicinal qualities along with binders to maintain the pill shape. The binders currently being used are usually sucrose (a natural form of sugar), the gum of a tree (Gum acacia), and potato starch. It is best to use these products intact, without excessive processing, because this can make them difficult to digest. In and of themselves, they are considered inert. Tablets also contain talc powder and magnesium stearate. These are needed to keep the tablets from sticking to the mold that forms them. They are present in tiny amounts and are considered completely safe. I, however, have a doubting mind and wonder about the long-term effect of such products. I prefer powders.

Due to my travel schedule in Europe and the varied locations in which I work, I find it more practical to have pharmacies in each country prepare my formulas. Then they are fresh, of high quality, and can be sent directly to the client. Because I work throughout Europe and England, this also saves me from having to carry around large quantities of plants, or tinctures and powders of plants. Naturally, the one that I do not have will be the one that I need for a client. While this approach may not suit some professionals, it works very well for self-care. However, it is always best to prepare your own formulas if possible.

For the first few years of my practice, I tried to use manufactured formulas. I found these to be generally unsatisfactory, not because of any fault in the retail formula, but because they seldom (if ever) fit the clients' individual needs. Although the general idea with manufactured formulas is that you can mix and match them to fit your clients' problems, I found that this method seldom matched my clients' pocketbooks. Nor was the idea of taking ten different pills twice or three times a day very appealing.

When I began to have specific formulas made for my clients on a regular basis, my rate of success greatly improved. It also provided fresh plants for the client and lowered the cost of treatment. The disadvantage was that powdered formulas generally taste bad, which is a problem for some people (usually the ones that would benefit the most from actually *tasting* bitter tastes). This was easily solved by having the herbalist or pharmacist put the powders into capsules of vegetable origin—"Veggie Caps," as they are called in the industry. Doses for powders vary from 4 to 8 grams per day. Powders have a short shelf life and must be stored correctly (i.e., in air-tight glass jars in the dark—as in a cupboard). They last anywhere from three to twelve months.

Using the whole plant is very effective in correcting long-standing imbalances of the doshas (humors), detoxifying the intestinal tract, correcting digestion, nourishing the nervous system, balancing the endocrine system, and blending all of these actions together should it be needed. Taking the whole plant allows the body's natural digestive enzymes to break down and assimilate the many active and inactive components in any given plant. It is the best method for long-term use, because powered plants are made of the water and earth elements—the basic elements of the body.

This approach has not been researched by modern medicine to any extent. It is, however, the basis of Ayurvedic and Chinese pharmacology, the two oldest existing medicinal systems. This is why I follow the rules of these two systems in my own formulations.

Another point to understand about the use of herbal powders is that they should be of *medicinal quality*. This does not mean a powder that you have ground up in your coffee grinder. Medicinal powders are very fine and do not have chunks or bits that can make you choke. In India, the powders are ground and sifted through a cloth several times. The leftovers can be used to make a tea. It is more practical to buy the plants in powdered form or to have your herbalist grind them for you. This is a decided disadvantage, but one more than worth the trouble.

If it is not possible for someone to grind the plants for you, you can use a coffee grinder and a strainer to sift the mix. Be prepared to spend a few hours grinding your formula. It is very important not to let your grinder overheat the herbs, as this can burn off valuable volatile oils.

Doses of powdered formulas vary from 2 to 4 grams twice a day, or 4 to 8 grams in total per day. A level teaspoon is about 2 grams (depending on which parts of the plants are used, since roots are heavier than leaves), a slightly rounded teaspoon is about 3 grams, and a heaping teaspoon is between 3.5 to 4.5 depending on your powder. Hence, an "average" teaspoon is about 3 grams.

I will not go into the medicinal qualities of the individual plants listed, or provide their Ayurvedic energetics. If this information is required or of interest to you, it is easily found in the classic, *Yoga of Herbs*,[1] by Drs. Frawley and Lad. This information is supplemented by Michael Tierra's two classic books, *Planetary Herbology* and *The Way of Herbs*.[2] These works have strongley influenced my use of herbs. In fact, these men are my teachers and, in a sense, my work is simply an individual adaptation of their innovative groundwork. Their books can be used as a resource for all

---

[1] Dr. David Frawley, and Dr. Vasant Lad, *The Yoga of Herbs* (Twin Lakes, WI: Lotus Press, 1986).

[2] Michael Tierra, *Planetary Herbology* (Twin Lakes, WI: Lotus Press, 1998) and *The Way of Herbs* (New York: Pocket Books, 1980).

the information presented in this book about herbs and plants in general.

To formulate a mixture of plants, I use one or several plants to form the primary action of the formula. I then use one or several plants to supplement or support this action. These supporting plants can also address other secondary issues in the body. Then I add digestives that increase the overall power of digestion and help the body to assimilate the formula. Along with the digestives, I try to make sure that one of the ingredients helps to eliminate toxins that may be liberated through the action of the primary and supporting herbs. Many times, I add a protective or harmonizing plant to balance the main direction of the formula. Generally, I add a stimulator to the formula to increase its potency—either ginger powder for vata and kapha or cinnamon for pitta, because these are easy to obtain.

My formulas thus consist of several different mechanisms:

Primary action;
Supporting action;
Eliminating action;
Protective or harmonizing action;
Digestive action;
Stimulant action.

One ingredient may support several of these actions. A single herb is not needed for each one.

In the formulas in Table 4 and the ones that follow, you will find a number in front of each herb. This indicates the ratio of the plant in the formula. I use this method instead of citing the number of grams because it is more flexible for calculating the amount you want to make. Most pharmacies or herbalists are familiar with this method.

Table 4. Sample Formula for a Therapeutic Powder

Dosha	(Ratio) Herb	Part of Plant	Effect on Metabolism	Effect on Dosha
Kapha	(3) Angelica	root	heating	+P
	(2) Agnus Castus	seed	heating	+P
	(2) Pennyroyal	plant	heating	+P (mildly)
	(2) Gotu Kola	plant	cooling	=VPK
	(1) Fenugreek	seed	heating	+P
	(1) Cumin	seed	cooling	=VPK
	(1) Ginger	root	heating	+P

In the example given in Table 4, the main herb is Angelica (3), then three supporting herbs are added (2), along with three digestive and stimulant herbs (1). If you total all the numbers given in parentheses, they equal 12. Now decide how much powder you want—perhaps 300 grams, enough for six to eight weeks, depending on the dose. Divide 300 by 12 (the total from the formula) and you have 25. This means that there will be 75 grams (25 X 3) of Angelic, 50 grams each of the supporting herbs (25 X 2), and 25 grams each of the digestive herbs and spices (25 X 1). If you want 600 grams total, divide 600 by 12 and you have a unit of 50 instead of 25, so the amount of each ingredient would be doubled.

While this may seem confusing to some (it is to me, as I am terrible at math!), it is actually a much better method, because it gives you complete freedom in deciding how much powder you want to buy at any given time. If everything is given in grams, it becomes tiresome to figure out different quantities. It is best never to buy more than what you can use in a six-month period. If you have easy access to herbs, three months is even better, because they will stay fresher. If you are on a limited budget, buy your herbs monthly. On the average, a formula will cost between $10 to $25 a month, depending on the type and quantity of herbs that are in it.

Table 4 also gives the classifications of each herb, which constitutional type the formula helps, the herb's amount, its common herb name (Latin names are given in Appendix 4), the part of the plant used, whether it stimulates the metabolism (heating) or lowers metabolic function (cooling), and the effect it has on the doshas. The letter given in the final column indicates the humor that will be aggravated by the sole use of the plant, not the overall effect of the formula. Each formula is designed to balance the humor for which it is given, Table 4 gives a formula for kapha. Therefore, it will be appropriate to balance kapha women.

Dual types can use the formula that corresponds to the aspect of their constitution that is being disturbed at the moment. For example, if you are a pitta/vata type and you are experiencing problems of nervousness (vata) along with other symptoms, choose the vata formula. Or if you are experiencing skin inflammation (pitta) with the same symptoms, choose the pitta formula. It is difficult to chose any "ready made" formula. The ones I give can be used as guidelines to adapt to your constitution. In this regard, the *Yoga of Herbs* is indispensable.

Ayurveda uses this basic method of compounding formulas because it was observed that, by using several plants that have a similar action, the result is much greater than just using any one of the same plants singularly. This is a science and requires much study and practice to perfect. The formulas that I give in this book are basic ones that can be built on and expanded. They also represent my approach and may not fit other practitioners. I have achieved excellent results in most cases. *It is most important to question who is taking the formula and whether this person has the ability to digest it, assimilate it and consistently take it.* This is important in self-care as well. I have put digestive spices in each formula to account for this point.

Readers should note that I work with several exceptions in regard to herbs. For example, I use the European and North American variety of angelica throughout this book instead of the Chinese variety, dong quai. I have used angelica with good success in Europe where dong quai is either unavailable or too expensive to use. If you have access to dong quai root that has been powdered (or your herbal store can do it for you), it is better for long-term use than the normal angelica. The Chinese variety has greater tonic properties and is considered to rejuvenate the reproductive organs. The European angelica has also been shown to have estrogenic effects, while dong quai has not shown these qualities. Also note that I have used barberry as a root. Very often it is sold as a root/bark combination and this is fine to use. Either may be used, depending on availability.

Please note that one plant is used several times in this book whose internal use is restricted in the United States—calamus root. This restriction is not in effect in continental Europe or in the United Kingdom. If used in small amounts, especially in conjunction with valerian root, it is the best nerve tonic and combination to balance the nervous aspect of the vata dosha. Its continuous use in Asia for thousands of years would seem to provide a substantial basis for a review by the FDA in the United States of its internal medical use in small amounts in blended formulas. In years of using it in Europe, I have yet to have a client complain of any negative side effect. Quite the contrary. The use of calamus in this book does not condone its use or contravene the decisions of the FDA. It acknowledges simply the Ayurvedic understanding of its traditional usage and my own clinical experience in Europe.

CHAPTER EIGHT

Depression

---

*Effort towards Realization is like the attempt to stamp with
one's foot on the shadow cast by one's head.
Effort will always make it recede.*

—Tripura Rahasya

Depression is a generic term that has become so broad as to
lose meaning—that is unless, of course, you are depressed!
There are two clear classifications of depression: biochemical
and mental.

Biochemical depression involves the endocrine system, of
which we spoke earlier, and relates to vata disturbances. This
category could be called a disease, as it is simply a disorder in
the endocrine function which, as we now know, affects the
whole body/mind state. Herbs work to correct this rather
easily. Personally, I hardly see this kind of depression as an illness, but rather as a lack of understanding about the body's
functions and signs. This will be clarified later. Depression of
mental origin, however, can become an illness if not addressed, but in reality it also is a question of ignorance.

To understand depression from a mental standpoint, it is
necessary to understand how the mind, emotions, and feelings function. Lack of knowledge about how our minds
function is called ignorance. Without this understanding,
the generic term "depression" cannot be understood or the
condition eliminated. The Ayurvedic understanding of the
mind has its origins in Vedic times more than 7,000 years
ago. Much of the information presented here comes from
the Upanishads, ancient scriptures found at the end of the
Vedas (books of knowledge).

The Vedic perspective is especially interesting for two reasons: the sages who perceived the workings of the mind where able to completely disassociate from it and thus had a truly objective view of its functions; and it works.

The primary mistake that people make is in not considering how the mind functions. They thus become trapped by thoughts, moods, and feelings that are transitory. These transient objects—thoughts, emotions, and feelings—are just that: transient. They pass through the field of conscious awareness in a continuous flow. One thing is certain about the mental function—it is always changing.

This is easily observable. Pick any thought that is going through your mind—the new shoes you saw in a shop window this morning—and try to hold onto it. Think of nothing other than the new shoes. Soon that thought will be replaced by another (is it gone already?). Your stomach will grumble, you will think about a handbag that matches the new shoes you saw, your child will call, or another thought will pass through your mind.

In the Ayurvedic sense, "mind" comprises thinking (movement of thought), intellectual reasoning, memory, emotions, and feelings. In Ayurvedic psychology, each of these has a specific name, but they all function together and so can simply be called the "mind." It is interesting to note that the emotions and feelings are considered so intrinsic to mental function they are not classified as being separate from the workings of the mind. Why is this?

What is it that perceives the emotion or feeling? When you say, "I am depressed," what is it that becomes aware of this state? When you say, "I feel bad" or "I feel good," what is it that contains an awareness of these passing states? By the same token, what is it that comprehends the thought of the new shoes passing by? Or the stomach rumbling? Or the needs of your child? Some process occurs that is not only conscious, but is also aware of what is passing—be it a thought, emotion, or feeling. This total functioning we call the "mind" or "mental field" in Ayurveda.

Normally, we do not question what passes through this mental field or mind. We are vaguely aware of thoughts or emotions crossing this field of conscious awareness. Occasionally, we grab onto one thought and follow it until it fizzles out. The mental perception is often so vague that people in general are not aware that there is not a continuous stream of thoughts, but rather many different individual thoughts passing separately. Figure 1 (page 86) shows how people normally see their minds.

The large thick line that is passing through the mental field (represented by the empty head) shows how we see the mind. All we are aware of is the seemingly solid, thick transference of thoughts, which we group together. Figure 2 (page 86) shows us, however, that, in reality, this solid mass of thoughts is nothing more than many individual thoughts or emotions passing through the field at great speed. Check this out for yourself right now. Pick a thought and hold on to it. Let it go and pick another one. Do this over and over again. Can you see that there really is no such a thing as "thinking," but rather that "thinking" is comprised of many different individual objects, thoughts, each one different than the other?

Depression, according to this explanation, occurs when a thought or emotion is chosen and then gets stuck in the mental field and won't go away. It stays inside and goes around and around, until we go mad, get stressed, get depressed, or have a nervous breakdown. Figure 3 (page 86) illustrates this. All mental troubles result from latching on to a single thought, emotion, or feeling and staying in a relationship with it. This prevents the natural flow of thoughts through the mental field.

What also becomes apparent in these figures is that you have a choice. You can pick any thought you like. Verify this. Is this true? Test it and see. Do you have the ability to choose and then release any thought that is passing through your mental field of awareness? When you have confirmed this fact, you have empowered yourself.

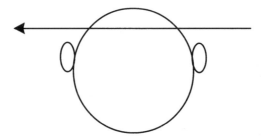

Figure 1.   Thinking, as commonly perceived.

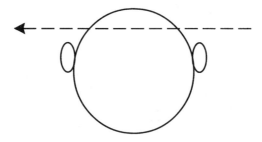

Figure 2.   Thinking, as perceived in Ayurveda.

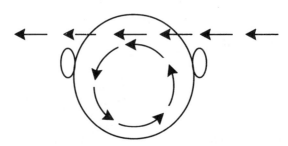

Figure 3.   Depression from an Ayurvedic perspective.

You have suddenly become the master, when seconds before you were the slave. This drastic shift of power results from a small but critical change. You now have the power to choose. You have always had that power, but you were only vaguely aware of it, or perhaps you were never aware of it. The lack of awareness of this choice enslaves you to anything that passes through your head, good or bad, happy or depressing. By choosing, you change your life, you take charge of your mind and emotions.

How you do this will depend on your personal affinities. Why did the thought of the new shoes come into your mental field instead of the thought of a new motorcycle? (Perhaps you wanted new boots for your motorcycle!) Each person has different affinities and attractions. These affinities cause certain feelings, emotions, and thoughts to be chosen by the consciousness.

Your affinites can be of two kinds. The first and most troublesome type of affinities come from conditioned behavior—what we learn from society, family, and friends. The second come from latent impressions that are either genetic or are carried from previous incarnations. In fact, both types are what are called latent impressions in Ayurveda, which gives two different names to distinguish between them. *Samskaras* are conditioned affinities that are picked up in this life, and *vasanas* are those impressions that are inherent in the human being.

Examples of the first are already clear: girls wear pink and boys wear blue. Stupid things like this (unless you like wearing pink) are drilled into us before we can hear or speak. "Girls like clothes and boys like cars." "You are stupid." "You are so bright." "You are beautiful, but so slow to . . ." And so we are conditioned, for better or worse.

The other kind of affinities are not as clear and are not at all understood by modern psychologists. The vasanas are very deep and lie in the unconscious and subconscious mind. The primary vasana is actually the source of the mind itself and of both the unconscious and subconscious minds.

The primary vasana is that "I am limited to the body." This gives rise to the whole physical and mental function. The vasanas of which we are semiconscious are the ones that propel us through life, making us lawyers, writers, artists, or housewives. These are strong, deep forces in life that can be seen simply as primal affinities that pull us toward different careers, persons,, and ideals.

Simply speaking, these two different kinds of affinities are what get us into relationships with the thoughts and emotions that are passing through the mental field. This is where problems begin and when we must assert our choice.

Neither the thoughts nor the emotions are problematic, but the relationship we have with them can be. These relationships are due to affinities that come from both conditioned behavior and from deep primal sources. The trick here is not to dwell on the reason for the affinities. This is the realm of psychotherapy and psychology. It is useful to a point, but limited in actually bringing peace of mind. It is useful to help understand the sources and causes of the conditionings. This, however, will seldom bring peace and contentment according to Ayurveda.

An example will be beneficial. I get depressed each time I feel my partner is becoming emotionally aggressive. I feel hurt and am unable to express my hurt. I also feel the aggression is unjustified, which adds to my frustration. Because I am unable to express this, I end up feeling depressed.

In this example, the depression is clearly the result of two factors, both of which stem from conditioned behavior. I have learned from my parents and family not only to accept emotional aggression, but not to express how I feel about it. To complicate matters, I have been taught to internalize these feelings until I become depressed by the whole matter. This is all conditioned behavior.

Instead of spending several thousand dollars to be able to write your parents hate mail—which can be helpful on a beginning level, provided you don't actually mail the letters—why not attack the root of the problem? Ayurveda feels that, instead of wasting a lot of time and money on peripheral issues, why not go directly to the primary issue, which is to cut the relationship with the conditioned behavior that creates the affinity?

I am the first one to admit that this method is not easy. It doesn't come in a box to which you just add water. I am also the first to attest to its efficiency. I am grateful for the years I spent in therapy, yet I am acutely aware of its limitations in actually bringing me peace—in eliminating depression. This method does work. It works with time and patience, because we have to relearn or change the habitual manner in which we have been taught to deal with things.

It is necessary to understand one other point before the whole Ayurvedic picture falls into place. We have seen that we have a choice, yet what is this choice? My teacher put it very simply and it is his advice that I still follow after years. Ask yourself if this activity, thought, emotion, or whatever, brings you peace. Or does it bring unhappiness and disturbances? By questioning ourselves like this, things become very simple—either a thought brings peace of mind, or it brings disturbance. Either an emotion is calming, or it is disruptive. Either an activity brings fulfillment, or it brings dissatisfaction.

We have the power to choose peace in our lives, or we have the power to choose misery. More often than not, we are conditioned to choose misery. Therefore, we must change our conditioning or mental habits. This takes some effort and time, but it is infinitely worthwhile.

Peace comes when we eliminate the activities that disturb it or prevent it from coming. Hence, we can see that, just by removing thoughts, emotions, or activities that disturb us, we can find happiness and eliminate moods like depression.

For example, I am depressed because I am alone and I have no one who loves me. The feeling of isolation is depressing to me. After some years, the pattern becomes clear:

when I think about it, I get very depressed for some weeks. The habit is clear and I can see that it is destructive, yet I continue.

To break out of this, first identify the actual thought that starts the relationship—"no one loves me." When the "no one loves me" thought comes into your mental field and you become aware of it, this is a critical moment. You have an instant in which to choose to let it go out of your head with the other thoughts. Simply recognize the thought. "Ah, yes, I know you, you make me depressed. I do not want to get into a relationship with you now." Choose this and divert your attention to something else. If your attention can be diverted with a firm decision, you have won and the thought will pass on. It may come back in a few minutes, or hours, or days. Then you must repeat these same steps over and over, until the thought finally gives up and leaves.

If I walk into a room where you are sitting and you ignore me, sooner or later I will get fed-up from waiting and I will leave. Thoughts are like this. If you give them attention, they will stay. If you divert your attention, they will become tired and leave—in time. Your ability to firmly and consistently divert your attention will indicate your level of success. Don't worry if you fall into the old pattern a few times because you could not catch it soon enough. And above all, don't use this method to self-criticize, because both positive and negative attention can feed thoughts and emotions.

Here is what to do if you fall into depression. Divert your attention, using one of two methods: physical activity (running or cleaning the house) and thought substitution. The physical substitute is easiest, but is usually effective only as long as you do the activity. Thought substitution is more effective, but requires more practice. The most effective substitutes are sounds.

There are several key sounds that are very useful because they vibrate at certain frequencies that have an effect on the nervous system. Different sounds are used for different needs. Below is a brief description of key sounds. More information can be found in Dr. Frawley's book,[1] from which this material is taken.

Hum (the "u" as in "put")—dispels fear and anxiety
Shrim ("shreem")—is cooling, creative, and feminine
Ram (the "a" as in "father")—is protecting, calm, and peaceful
Sham ("shum")—brings detachment, peace, and contentment

Vata types can best benefit from Ram and Hum. Pitta types may benefit best from the use of Shrim and Sham. Kapha people will do well with Hum. Any of the three constitutions can use these sounds as needed. They generally succeed best if they are used for a period of time and not just when you are in a depression.

The use of sound is very effective in balancing vata and all forms of vata mental disturbances, like depression. These sounds are very good preventive measures if you are prone to chronic bouts of depression. Do not wait until you are depressed to use these sounds—they will help somewhat, but that effect will be much greater if you learn to use them before depression sets in. Experiment with the sounds and find one that you like. At first, pronounce the sound that you choose aloud, until it is clear in your mind. Then use it silently. This way, you can use it in public and no one will be aware that you have substituted a sound for a disturbing thought.

Ayurveda states that the use of these sounds is the most effective. There are other sounds as well, and you may use anything you wish. The main point is to divert the attention. This should be understood. There is nothing magical or mysterious about the mind and its functioning. If you use

[1] Dr. David Frawley, *Ayurvedic Healing: A Comprehensive Guide* (Sandy, UT: Passage Press, 1989).

the word soap, soap, soap, it will serve to substitute the habitually disruptive thought. However, it is clear that we should learn from the experience of the ancients and use their suggestions. My own experience is that the sounds given above are very effective. In summary, we can perceive the mind in the following manner:

Thoughts are emotions and feelings, as well as ideas or objects.

Thoughts are individual things that we can accept or reject.

We have a fundamental choice.

This choice can be clarified by choosing either peaceful or disturbing experiences in the mental field.

Certain thoughts are troublesome because we have affinities for them.

Affinities are latent impressions of two kinds—conditioned and primal.

Our relationship with our affinities causes thoughts to become stuck in our mental field, causing depression.

The moment a thought becomes recognized, we can choose to let it go by making a firm choice for peace.

If we realize too late and become trapped in mental agitation, we can divert our attention by two means: physical activity or thought substitution.

Specific sounds are very effective in substituting thoughts, because they effect the nervous system through the vata dosha.

Substituting a thought with a sound should be practiced regularly throughout the day to be really effective.

This is a practical method for addressing mental disturbances of all kinds, not only depression. It can totally eliminate depression from your life. The key to using it is to understand clearly how your mind functions. Detach yourself from it. You are not limited to the mind and the mental field. You have a soul and other subtle aspects and can perceive your mind as a good servant and helper, which it is.

Mind becomes destructive in the role of the master. Observe how you have given away your power and become a slave to your mind and emotions. Enjoy the mind and emotions, but do not mistake them for yourself. They belong to you and, as such, you can dictate what you want to keep in your mind. This is the beginning of freedom.

The other cause of depression is a chemical imbalance in the endocrine system. The biggest problem with this kind of disorder is that it can lead to mental disturbance or depression through a lack of understanding. This is the primary problem. In and of itself, it is not difficult to correct. It is the damage that one can project on oneself that can be the most harmful.

Simple misunderstanding can lead you to view a chemical problem in the body as a personal shortcoming. The statement, "I am depressed" highlights this clearly. Are you really depressed or is it just a chemical imbalance in the body? If it is just in the body, can you really state, "I am depressed"? Isn't it more accurate to say, "The body is disturbed and is affecting my moods"?

In fact, this is the case. Unfortunately, we are not taught the real situation. We are programmed to think that whatever happens to the body is happening to us and is somehow our responsibility. If you cut your finger you say, "I cut *my* finger." If your body is out of balance for some reason, you say, "I am depressed." Both are things happening to the body. Both from external sources. The endocrine system does not just arbitrarily go out of balance. It needs external input to disrupt its functioning. Yes, this is true for your cycle as a woman as well. It is indicative of imbalance, not lack of health.

This biochemical disturbance can be caused by a number of factors. The main causes are those that disturb vata. This means the mind and the nervous system. Mental stress, lack of love, anxiety, fear, worry, and the overstimulation of the senses are the main external factors that disrupt the endocrine system. Internal factors include the ingestion of foods or products that have estrogenic chemicals, and medications of any kind.

As our whole food chain is filled with estrogenic chemicals, this alone is enough to disrupt the biochemical function of half of all the women in the United States. Many of these women will suffer depression as a symptom of having ingested these chemicals. A look at how many women take birth control pills gives an idea how many may have endocrine functions that are affected by the regular and prolonged use of these products.

Regardless whether the imbalance comes from mental or physical sources the result is the same—a disruption in the mind or body due to endocrine malfunction. It is not the purpose of this book to dwell on these aspects, but rather to point them out as a reality of our culture and times. When seen objectively, the occurrence of chronic, or monthly, bouts of depression can almost be taken as "normal," given the circumstances in which we live. We can, however, do something about it.

Before I give the practical methods of correction, I should point out that disassociating yourself from the chemical malfunction of your body can bring enormous freedom. It allows you to see that, in fact, nothing is wrong with *you*. You are fine and should not allow yourself to be categorized or put into a box as "unstable," "depressive," "oversensitive," "disturbed," etc. These labels do not allow you to be happy, nor do you have to accept them. You must, however, do something to get your body back in balance. This may be facilitated by using any of the methods that I described above for mental depression—especially if you have actually convinced yourself that something is wrong with you.

The best method for correcting the physical imbalance of the endocrine system is the use of a balanced herbal formula. This has a better effect than using one plant alone, because the doshas can be balanced at the same time.

St. John's Wort is a plant that has recently enjoyed a lot of publicity. It is very effective in helping the endocrine system find a balance. Many people find their depression cleared after using St. John's Wort. This supports the idea that there are indeed two distinct classes of depression—biochemical and mental. However, what is not commonly known is that prolonged use of St. John's Wort can be disruptive to the vata dosha and can cause it to imbalance if taken for long periods.

For this reason, a formula should be made according to your constitution. Table 5 gives several examples of formulas that I use for depression.

Table 5. Formulas for Treating Depression

Dosha	(Ratio) Herb	Part of Plant	Effect on Metabolism	Effect on Dosha
Vata	(3) St. John's Wort	plant	cooling	+V
	(2) Cramp Bark	bark	heating	+P
	(2) Agnus Castus	seed	heating	+P
	(2) Valerian	root	heating	+P
	(1) Calamus Root*	root	heating	+P
	(1) Fennel	seed	cooling	=VPK
	(1) Cumin	seed	cooling	=VPK
	(1) Ginger	root	heating	+P
Pitta	(3) St. John's Wort	plant	cooling	+V
	(2) Angelica	root	heating	+P
	(2) Agnus Castus	seed	heating	+P
	(2) Gotu Kola	plant	cooling	=VPK
	(1) Fennel	seed	cooling	=VPK
	(1) Cumin	seed	cooling	=VPK
	(1) Cinnamon	bark	heating	+P
Kapha	(3) St. John's Wort	plant	cooling	+V
	(2) Angelica	root	heating	+P
	(2) Agnus Castus	seed	heating	+P
	(2) Gotu Kola	plant	cooling	=VPK
	(1) Fenugreek	seed	heating	+P
	(1) Cumin	seed	cooling	=VPK
	(1) Ginger	root	heating	+P

*Internal use is currently restricted by the FDA in the United States.

Notice that each formula uses the same main plant, St. John's Wort, to balance the endocrine system. It is then supported by other plants to balance specific aspects of the endocrine function. Progesterone imbalance has been linked to all kinds of emotional disturbances, and agnus castus is the best plant available in the West to regulate it. Another supporting endocrine herb is used to balance the formula for the individual constitution type. Then a nervine is used to support the brain and nervous system (the choice depends on the constitution). Finally, several digestives are used to support the digestion and assimilation of the formula and to treat the digestive tract in general. Remember that there is no final word here, but rather use these formulas as a guide. *If vata is part of your constitution, I suggest that you use the vata formula.*

Case History 1

A woman, age 39, came to me for depression, nervousness, and mood swings from which she had suffered for several months. She had a vata/pitta constitution. Her *vikruti* (imbalanced state) showed both excessive vata and pitta. She had some digestive trouble in the small intestine and liver. She also had weak kidneys. She had a history of alcohol addiction and depression. I prescribed a simple formula due to the weakness of her liver (from years as an alcoholic):

Table 6. Formula for Case History 1

DOSHA	(RATIO) HERB	PART OF PLANT	EFFECT ON METABOLISM	EFFECT ON DOSHA
Vata/ **Pitta**	(3) St. John's Wort	plant	cooling	PK-V+
	(3) Gotu Kola	plant	cooling	KPV=
	(2) Gentian	root	cooling	PK-V+
	(2) Licorice	root	cooling	VP-K+
	(1) Calamus˙	root	heating	VK-P+
	(1) Ginger	root	heating	VK-P+

Dose: 3 grams of powder in warm water with natural sugar twice a day, taken between meals.

˙ Internal use is currently restricted by the FDA in the United States.

Within seven days she felt better. After ten days, she was 50 percent improved. In two weeks, she called to thank me saying she felt "normal" again and amazed that months of feeling badly had been cured so quickly. She continued the treatment for six weeks and used it over the next year when under stress. She changed her work and is feeling much better and happier.

Her formula was simple, using only one digestive (gentian) to support the weak liver and small intestine. The addition of licorice to support the kidneys and to help harmonize the whole formula was especially important because she was also prone to imbalance with high pitta problems.

CHAPTER NINE

Premenstrual and Menstrual Difficulties

Moksha (liberation) is not anything to be got afresh for it is already there only to be realized. Such realization arises with the elimination of igno-rance. Absolutely nothing more is required to achieve the aim of life.

—Tripura Rahasya

According to Ayurveda, all menstrual difficulties are related in some way to an imbalance in the vata dosha. Most origi-nate from a disruption in the function of vata. All treatments should begin with an assessment of the state of the vata hu-mor in the body.

The tongue provides a good indication of the state of vata in the body generally and in the internal organs espe-cially. The constitution of the person should be determined first. The tongue can give indications of constitution as ex-plained earlier (see page 17). Disturbed vata may appear on the tongue as roughness, cracks, pimples, and brownish coatings. If the tongue trembles, this may also indicate an imbalance in vata.

Other indications in the body are intestinal gas, bloat-ing, migrating pain, irregularity in digestion or menstrua-tion, twitching body parts, nervous disorders, internal or external dryness, brittle hair, dull skin or hair, sharp pains, and any mental agitation such as stress or nervousness. If the mind is unable to stay focused, this indicates an imbalance of vata. If the person is talking excessively or too fast, it is also indicative of a vata nature or imbalanced vata.

Next, see if any other humor is involved in the symptoms or root cause. Then a history should be noted: what, where, how long, when in the cycle, and the resulting feeling or symptom that comes with it. Write this information down and clarify the whole situation as this will help you to establish a therapeutic approach. Remember, even a slight discomfort or mood swing is indicative of an imbalance in Ayurveda and should be remedied as soon as possible.

Next, address the tissue levels and systems involved. This can help to further pinpoint a treatment approach (see chapter 3). Finally, consider the organs involved in the symptoms or root causes. The health of the organs comes from the proper digestion and development of the tissue levels. If this process is disturbed, the organs can malfunction. Other determining factors include those stemming from ignorance, or what we might call bad choices, like drinking too much alcohol or too many soft drinks. These influences can disrupt organ function, and can also imbalance the tissues and systems associated with them. Hence, the focus on individual organs is the last consideration, but is still important.

Now you are ready to address the symptoms. If they are minor or not too difficult, it is best to ignore them or bear them for a cycle or two, if possible, giving the formula time to work. If, however, the problems are acute, some additional steps should be taken immediately, in addition to those that work to correct the chronic cause. Symptoms (short of an infection) seldom appear suddenly. Even infections generally need a supportive environment in the body to take root. Look carefully to determine whether you have been unhappy or disturbed recently, as this is a major factor in disruptions to the endocrine system, and so to your monthly cycle.

At this point, it is worth mentioning the effect of unsatisfying sexual relationships. Tension around sexual intercourse is one important cause of endocrine disturbance. It is my observation that this is often due to a lack of love. It may be that, although the love is there, the woman does not feel that the man loves her. This is a deep subject with no simple answer or remedy. It is important to look and see if you do feel loved or if you feel used. The general feeling of being used will cause vata to be disturbed and can give rise to many menstrual problems. If love is not present at all in the relationship, you can expect a number of health problems at some point. A loving, caring relationship is a good cure for many health problems.

Premenstrual Difficulties

Premenstrual problems are almost always caused by a disturbance in the vata dosha, which can go on to derange the function of the other two doshas. If vata is solely responsible for the symptoms, they will be irregular and unpredictable. They may be strongest during the vata times of the day—sunrise and sunset. If pitta is involved, inflammations of the vagina or skin may occur, along with frustration, irritability, and anger. Sweating and sudden temperature changes may occur. Symptoms will be strongest during the middle of the day and at midnight—pitta times.

When kapha becomes involved, heaviness, tiredness, and lethargy are common. You will tend to internalize your emotions and become sentimental. Fluid retention is a classic characteristic of kapha disturbed by a vata imbalance. Symptoms will be strongest in the morning and evening—the time of kapha. Dual constitutions may experience a blend of these symptoms. Premenstrual problems, however, are usually more indicative of an imbalanced state (vikruti) than they are of the natal constitution (prakruti). The only sure way to know is to see an Ayurvedic practitioner.

You will notice that a number of herbs are used over and over to treat the different symptoms of premenstrual problems. These main combinations have proven effective over time in treating all kinds of troubles associated with menstruation and premenstrual difficulties. Small changes are made here and there to adjust the formulas to fit the different constitutional types and specific problems more accurately.

Headaches

Headaches can arise from two distinct sources: one digestive and one hormonal. This treatment approach is based on the latter, a hormonal disturbance of premenstrual origin, assuming that it is the kind of headache that comes with your monthly cycle. The idea here is that pitta (which controls the blood) becomes disturbed by the aggravation of vata. The treatment first tries to balance vata and then treats pitta, the actual cause of the blood vessels becoming dilated and pressing on the nerves, thereby causing pain.

The vata channel (vayu nadis or srota) is congested, blocking both apana and prana vayu. This in turn upsets the blood channel that is feeding the blood dhatu. The vayu is pushing on the channel, not the dhatu. Using herbs that clear the apana and prana channels is the first line of treatment. The next is to stimulate the blood channel.

Symptomatically chrysanthemum flowers can be used to treat headaches. Infuse 2 teaspoons of dried flowers in a cup of water. Drink one or two cups. This pacifies pitta and reduces the headache pain. See Table 7 for formulas for treating headaches.

Table 7. Formulas for Treating Headaches

Dosha	(Ratio) Herb	Part of Plant	Effect on Metabolism	Effect on Dosha
Vata	(3) Angelica	root	heating	+P
	(2) Pennyroyal	plant	heating	+P (mildly)
	(2) Agnus Castus	seed	heating	+P
	(2) Gotu Kola	plant	cooling	=VPK
	(1) Fenugreek	seed	heating	+P
	(1) Cumin	seed	cooling	=VPK
	(1) Ginger	root	heating	+P

Dose: 1 teaspoon (approx. 3 gr.) twice a day with warm water and honey between meals.

Table 7. Formulas for Treating Headaches (cont.)

Pitta	(3) Gotu Kola	plant	cooling	=VPK
	(2) Pennyroyal	plant	heating	+P (mildly)
	(2) Angelica	root	heating	+P
	(2) Agnus Castus	seed	heating	+P
	(1) Cumin	seed	cooling	=VPK
	(1) Fennel	seed	cooling	=VPK
	(1) Cinnamon	bark	heating	+P

Dose: 1 teaspoon (approx. 3 gr.) twice a day with warm water and natural sugar between meals.

Kapha	(3) Angelica	root	heating	+P
	(2) Agnus Castus	seed	heating	+P
	(2) Pennyroyal	plant	heating	+P (mildly)
	(2) Gotu Kola	plant	cooling	=VPK
	(1) Fenugreek	seed	heating	+P
	(1) Cumin	seed	cooling	=VPK
	(1) Ginger	root	heating	+P

Dose: 1 teaspoon (approx. 3 gr.) twice a day with warm water and honey between meals.

Doses for the above formulas can vary from 4 to 8 grams per day (2 X 2 gr. or 2 X 4 gr.), taken between meals with warm water for two to four months, depending on the person and how long the problem has existed.

Case History 2

A 38-year-old woman came to me with many premenstrual problems, including very irregular cycles and very strong headaches before her menstruation. She had a pitta constitution, and a very responsible job, and was married. Both vata and pitta were imbalanced. She had taken the pill for over ten years. She had toxins present of a fire nature (pitta). These needed to be cleared and her digestive system needed to be balanced. I suggested the formula shown in Table 8 (see page 104).

Table 8. Formula for Case History 2

DOSHA	(RATIO) HERB	PART OF PLANT	EFFECT ON METABOLISM	EFFECT ON DOSHA
Pitta	(3) Angelica	root	heating	+P
	(3) Agnus Castus	seed	heating	+P
	(3) Gentian	root	cooling	+V
	(3) Burdock	root	cooling	+V
	(2) Valerian	root	heating	+P
	(2) Licorice	root	cooling	+K
	(1) Cumin	seed	cooling	=VPK
	(1) Cinnamon	bark	heating	+P

Dose: 3 grams of powder twice per a with warm water and natural sugar before meals.

I suggested she stop taking the pill. I attributed much of her problem to a chronic imbalance of vata (which moved up to increase pitta), caused, in part, by her long-term use of the pill. In a month, her symptoms were much better. By the third month, they had cleared and her cycle was regular, though longer. It took six months before she was completely healthy with a regular cycle, although her headaches had been gone since the second month. She is now the happy mother of a beautiful baby girl, has changed her job and her house, and has decided to keep her husband.

Case History 3

A 38-year-old woman came to me because she wanted to lose weight, was tired all the time, was very nervous, and was experiencing strong headaches two days before each menstruation. She was a vata/kapha type with an imbalance of vata. I suggested the formula shown in Table 9 (see page 105).

Table 9. Formula for Case History 3

Dosha	(Ratio) Herb	Part of Plant	Effect on Metabolism	Effect on Dosha
Vata/	(3) Angelica	root	heating	+P
Kapha	(3) Gentian	root	cooling	+V
	(2) Agnus Castus	seed	heating	+P
	(2) Black Cohosh	root	cooling	+V
	(2) Burdock	root	cooling	+V
	(2) Turmeric	root	heating	=VPK
	(2) Barberry	root	heating	+V
	(1) Fenugreek	seed	heating	+P
	(1) Fennel	seed	cooling	=VPK
	(1) Cumin	seed	cooling	=VPK
	(1) Cinnamon	bark	heating	+P
	(1) Ginger	root	heating	+P

Dose: 3.5 grams of powder twice a day with warm water and honey before meals.

She had a digestive problem in the small intestines that needed to be addressed with gentian root. Her whole metabolism was slow and slightly toxic, hence the need to use the turmeric-barberry combination to remove the toxins and promote digestion. Her problems cleared in three months and she lost a few pounds.

Cramps and Pain

Cramps and pain indicate an imbalance in the vata dosha and relate directly to the apana vayu. They are a result of vata constriction and are more prone to happen in vata types or vata dual constitutions. Treatment tends to be long-term, since the formulas work to balance vata in the constitution. This disorder involves both the apana and vyana vayus in the vayu channel (prana srota). The menstruation channel will be disturbed by this and can affect pitta via this srota. Excess kapha can constrict vata as well by moving from the plasma channel into the vayu channel, creating pressure and blockage. Immediate relief can be had by taking 2 teaspoons of black haw (Viburnum prunifolium) bark and infusing them in a cup of hot water. Drink one or two cups twice per day while cramps last. Formulas for treating cramps and pain are shown in Table 10.

Table 10. Formulas for Treating Cramps and Pain

Dosha	(Ratio) Herb	Part of Plant	Effect on Metabolism	Effect on Dosha
Vata	(3) Cramp Bark	bark	heating	+P
	(2) Angelica	root	heating	+P
	(2) Agnus Castus	seed	heating	+P
	(2) Mugwort	plant	heating	+P
	(2) Valerian	root	heating	+P
	(1) Fennel	seed	cooling	=VPK
	(1) Ginger	root	heating	+P
Dose: 1 teaspoon (approx. 3 gr.) twice a day with warm water and honey between meals.				
Pitta	(3) Cramp Bark	bark	heating	+P
	(2) Agnus Castus	seed	heating	+P
	(2) Black Cohosh	root	cooling	+V
	(2) Mugwort	plant	heating	+P
	(2) Licorice	root	cooling	+K
	(1) Fennel	seed	cooling	=VPK
	(1) Cinnamon	bark	heating	+P
Dose: 1 teaspoon (approx. 3 gr.) twice a day with warm water and natural sugar between meals.				
Kapha	(3) Cramp Bark	bark	heating	+P
	(3) Angelica	root	heating	+P
	(2) Agnus Castus	seed	heating	+P
	(2) Dandelion	root	cooling	+V
	(1) Fenugreek	seed	heating	+P
	(1) Cumin	seed	cooling	=VPK
	(1) Ginger	root	heating	+P
Dose: 1 teaspoon (approx. 3 gr.) twice a day with warm water and honey between meals.				

Doses for the above formulas vary from 4 to 8 grams per day (2 X 2 gr. or 2 X 4 gr.), taken between meals with warm water for two to four months, depending on the person and how long the problem has existed. The longer the problem has persisted, the longer you will have to take this formula.

Case History 4

A 32-year-of-old woman came to me with many problems, of which PMS was primary. She had much pain with her cycle, as well as headaches. Her constitution was kapha/pitta, with an imbalance of vata. Her symptoms included chronic constipation, weak kidneys, hay fever, and stress. Food tends to come up when we are stressed, so she had difficulty with digestion in general. She had some pitta toxins in the colon, low digestive ability (i.e., low *agni*) and malabsorption syndrome. I suggested the formula shown in Table 11.

Table 11. Formula for Case History 4

DOSHA	(RATIO) HERB	PART OF PLANT	EFFECT ON METABOLISM	EFFECT ON DOSHA
Kapha/ Pitta	(3) Agnus Castus	seed	heating	+P
	(3) Cramp Bark	bark	heating	+P
	(3) Barberry	root	heating	+V
	(2) Turmeric	root	heating	=VPK
	(2) Gentian	root	cooling	+V
	(2) Uva ursi	leaf	cooling	+V
	(2) Licorice	root	cooling	+K
	(1) Cardamom	seed	heating	+P
	(1) Fenugreek	seed	heating	+P
	(1) Fennel	seed	cooling	=VPK
	(1) Cumin	seed	cooling	=VPK
	(1) Ginger	root	heating	+P

Dose: 3.5 grams of powder twice a day with warm water and honey before meals.

After a few weeks, her digestion improved and her constipation disappeared. After two months, she felt better in her body in general, her cycle had improved slightly, and her stomach problems where gone. Although the level of stress in her life increased, her pain was minimal, yet not gone, after six months. This is an example of how lifestyle (increase of stress rather than a reduction) did not support the herbs enough, resulting in partial relief. The patient was happy, however, with even a partial cure.

Case History 5

Another 38-year-old woman came to me (they all seem to be 38 in these examples!) with general premenstrual problems. Pain and nervousness were her primary symptoms. She was a vata type, with an imbalance of vata. She was in generally good health, but had a chronically high level of vata and a life-history of premenstrual difficulties. I suggested the following formula shown in Table 12.

Table 12. Formula for Case History 5

DOSHA	(RATIO) HERB	PART OF PLANT	EFFECT ON METABOLISM	EFFECT ON DOSHA
Vata	(3) Cramp Bark	bark	heating	+P
	(3) Agnus Castus	seed	heating	+P
	(3) Angelica	root	heating	+P
	(2) European Madder	root	cooling	+V
	(2) Licorice	root	cooling	+K
	(2) Cardamom	seed	heating	+P
	(2) Fennel	seed	cooling	=VPK
	(1) Ginger	root	heating	+P
Dose: 2 "00" capsules* twice a day between meals.				

* Note: "0" capsules hold about 450 mgs of herbs and "00" capsules hold about 750 mgs.

It took almost six months, but all her premenstrual problems disappeared. She is a highly strung, active individual. As long as she maintains her equilibrium, she will stay well.

I do not subscribe to the new premenstrual syndrome (PMS) classifications that are becoming increasingly common in the medical community. Of course, Ayurveda does not consider these classifications uselful, since the traditional system is more comprehensive and offers a deeper insight into why these problems exist to begin with. I have, however, included a formula for each of the four categories, with an explanation based in Ayurvedic logic. Remember, I do not subscribe to this kind of symptomatic classification or symptomatic treatment. I include these only to help those who may not be comfortable using the Ayurvedic model.[1] Formulas for treating these symptoms are found in Table 13 (see page 110). All types of premenstrual problems should also be treated with diet. Chapter 14 looks at this topic in some depth.

PMS(A) is a vata imbalance with a pitta disturbance that occurs in some women. This can affect the prana vayu and the samana vayu. Nervines are needed to harmonize prana vayu. The best anti-vata herb combination is valerian and calamus. The digestion needs to be addressed, as pitta often becomes disturbed due to the chronic agitation of vata.

PMS(C) is a vata imbalance that affects the kidney/adrenal function and pancreas via the endocrine system. It relates primarily to the samana and apana vayus. This aggravates both pitta and kapha. Vata increases and moves into the small intestine, disrupting the function of agni and aggravating pitta. This, in turn, imbalances the pancreatic function

---

[1] I also must confess that I dislike the term PMS, which seems to me to turn a woman into a disease. Admittedly, I am oversensitive to classifications (which is why I practice Ayurveda) and so my opinion may not be of value. I have intentionally avoided using common words like PMS, period, etc., as they have negative connotations for many people, but here I will use the standard classifications.

and kapha. The blood (pitta) serves as a vehicle for the irritated kapha and pitta. Vata should be treated first, then pitta, and finally kapha. Toxins will most likely be present.

PMS(D) can be seen as a vata imbalance and relates primarily to the prana vayu. This imbalance is more indicative of an overall imbalance of the endocrine system, which is controlled by the prana vayu. Balancing the prana is the key in this treatment. This explains why it is often related to PMS(A).

PMS(H) is related to vata moving into the kapha dosha. The primary problem is the apana vayu disrupts the ovarian function and moves upward through the nervous system and vayu channels (prana srota) to the breasts and lymphatic system (controlled by kapha). Both vata and kapha must be addressed.

Table 13. Formulas for PMS Types

DOSHA	(RATIO) HERB	PART OF PLANT	EFFECT ON METABOLISM	EFFECT ON DOSHA
PMS(A)	(3) Agnus Castus	seed	heating	+P
	(2) Mugwort	plant	heating	+P
	(2) Angelica	root	heating	+P
	(2) Licorice	root	cooling	+K
	(2) Valerian	root	heating	+P
	(2) Turmeric	root	heating	=VPK
	(1) Calamus root *	root	heating	+P
	(1) Fennel	seed	cooling	=VPK
	(1) Ginger	root	heating	+P
Dose: 5–8 grams a day with warm water and natural sugar.				
PMS(C)	(3) Agnus Castus	seed	heating	+P
	(3) St. John's Wort	plant	cooling	+V
	(2) Angelica	root	heating	+P
	(2) Barberry **	root	heating	+V
	(2) Turmeric	root	heating	=VPK

Table 13. Formulas for PMS Types (cont.)

PMS(C) (cont.)	(2) Gentian**	root	cooling	+V
	(2) Dandelion	root	cooling	+V
	(2) Nettles	plant	cooling	+V
	(1) Licorice	root	cooling	+K
	(1) Fennel	seed	cooling	=VPK
	(1) Cumin	seed	cooling	=VPK
	(1) Ginger	root	heating	+P

Dose: 5–8 grams a day with warm water and natural sugar.

PMS(D)	(3) Dong Quai	root	heating	+P
	(3) St. John's Wort	plant	cooling	+V
	(2) Black Cohosh	root	cooling	+V
	(2) Agnus Castus	seed	heating	+P
	(2) Licorice	root	cooling	+K
	(2) Valerian	root	heating	+P
	(1) Calamus Root*	root	heating	+P
	(1) Fennel	seed	cooling	=VPK
	(1) Ginger	root	heating	+P

Dose: 5–8 grams a day with warm water and natural sugar.

PMS(H)	(3) Agnus Castus	seed	heating	+P
	(3) Angelica	root	heating	+P
	(2) Echinacea	root	cooling	+V
	(2) Barberry**	root	heating	+V
	(2) Turmeric	root	heating	=VPK
	(2) Dandelion	root	cooling	+V
	(2) Nettles	plant	cooling	+V
	(1) Fenugreek	seed	heating	+P
	(1) Ginger	root	heating	+P

Dose: 5–7 grams a day with warm water and a little honey.

*   Internal use is currently resrticted by the FDA in the United States
** If toxins are not present then the barberry and gentian can be eliminated.

Menstrual Difficulties

Menstrual problems trouble almost every woman during the course of her life. This section may not be very helpful for stopping acute irritations immediately (although that will also be addressed), but it will certainly provide an insight into why these problems have occurred and give some advice on how to prevent them from recurring.

Many of the herbs used here are the same as those used above, although the combinations may be somewhat different. It is important to remember that Ayurveda always treats your constitution. This may require the use of plants that are not considered to be directly beneficial for women. They are, however, beneficial for you as a person.

Ayurveda views menstrual problems as a combination of several factors. The vata dosha is of primary importance, followed by the pitta dosha. The vata moves through the vayu channel, therefore, obstructions or pressure on these channels will affect menstruation. Pitta moves through the blood and menstruation channels. Toxic blood conditions, caused by toxins in the digestive system, will move into the menstruation channel, thereby causing problems.

In addition, if either the plasma dhatu (kapha) or the blood dhatu are not correctly nourished, menstruation will be difficult. Poor plasma dhatu directly affects menstruation, because it is a subdhatu of plasma. Any problem in the plasma/lymphatic system will cause either deficient or excessive menstruation.

The blood dhatu is affected by the problems of the plasma dhatu and by digestive toxins. Poor liver function is not so much a cause of toxic blood as the outcome of a toxic digestive system that affects the blood, causing eventual liver congestion and failure. As the pitta dosha controls both the blood srota and the menstruation srota, an undernourished blood dhatu can precipitate chronic and hard-to-heal menstrual problems. Of course, the plasma dhatu must first be deficient for the blood dhatu to become deficient.

Tampons can be an important factor in your overall health. There is substantial proof that tampons are related to Toxic Shock Syndrome in some women. Studies show that a wood-fiber product that is used in the manufacturing of tampons is bleached with a product called dioxin, a by-product of chlorine bleaching and a known carcinogen. Why on Earth any one in their right mind would use such a product in the vagina just for aesthetics (a whiter white) is beyond human comprehension. Dioxin accumulates in fat tissues and has been linked to cancer, endrometriosis, and immune suppression. Who knows what else it may cause!

Rayon has also been linked to TSS, so if you use tampons, it is best to use all-cotton, nonbleached products. When I showed this study to my wife she chose not to use tampons any more; instead she uses pads. Health food stores do carry all-natural pads and tampons. In 1980, thirty-eight women died of tampon-related disease (TSS) in the United States. The Environmental Protection Agency did a study in 1994 that showed that 1 in every 1000 cases of cancer may be caused by dioxin—and the figure could be much higher than that. If you are having any kind of chronic menstrual problem, this may be a good place to begin looking for its cause. In addition, if you are trying to become pregnant and are having difficulties, you should know that dioxin has also been linked to low sperm counts in men. These chemicals remain in the body, and they are capable of affecting your partner as well.

It must be stressed that general good health is the best foundation for a trouble-free cycle; bad health is going to affect your menstruation. In this context, regular physical exercise and good food play an important role. It is naive to believe that taking herbs and not exercising or eating well will bring you health. Your overall lifestyle should be adjusted in conjunction with using these formulas. These formulas can help balance your overall health and the doshas that are behind your symptoms, but they may not reduce an acute symptom immediately.

Amenorrhea
(delay or absence of menstruation)

The following treatments are not for amenorrhea caused by diabetes or chronic wasting diseases. Since problems of the liver can also cause amenorrhea for pitta types, the blood and liver channels (ranjaka pitta) should become the focus of the treatment. It is also not for pubescent girls who have not had their first menstruation and are therefore classified as suffering from "primary" amenorrhea. For cases of primary amenorrhea, it is important for the mother to look closely at the home environment and see if there is some emotional disturbance that is preventing the beginning of normal menstruation.

Ayurveda sees amenorrhea as a constriction of the apana vayu and the vayu channel. The prana vayu may be involved, if there is a hormone imbalance. The constriction of the apana will stop the flow of pitta in the menstruation srota. While promoting blood flow is important, herbs that move the apana vayu should be the main focus. You should also try to determine why vata (apana vayu) has become disturbed in the first place.

Immediate relief can be brought about by a number of different plants. Tincture of myrrh (20 drops, four times a day) is effective. A tea of fresh ginger and pennyroyal, in equal amounts, is also a simple and effective remedy.

In the formulas in Table 14 (see page 115), dong quai is substituted for angelica, as it is thought to be better-suited and more specific for this kind of problem. These formulas are recommended for both chronic and irregular types of amehorrhea. Doses vary from 6–8 grams per day, (2 X 3 gr. or 2 X 4 gr.), taken between meals with warm water or ginger tea for two to four months, depending on how long the problem has existed.

Table 14. Formulas for Treating Amenorrhea

Dosha	(Ratio) Herb	Part of Plant	Effect on Metabolism	Effect on Dosha
Vata	(3) Dong Quai	root	heating	+P (mildly)
	(2) Agnus Castus	seed	heating	+P
	(2) Pennyroyal	plant	heating	+P (mildly)
	(2) Mugwort	plant	heating	+P
	(2) Turmeric	root	heating	=VPK
	(2) Licorice	root	cooling	+K
	(1) Fennel	seed	cooling	=VPK
	(1) Cumin	seed	cooling	=VPK
	(1) Ginger	root	heating	+P

Dose: 1 teaspoon (approx. 3 gr.) twice a day with warm water and honey between meals.

Dosha	(Ratio) Herb	Part of Plant	Effect on Metabolism	Effect on Dosha
Pitta	(3) Dong Quai	root	heating	+P (mildly)
	(2) Agnus Castus	seed	heating	+P
	(2) Raspberry	plant	cooling	+V
	(2) Dandelion	root	cooling	+V
	(2) Turmeric	root	heating	=VPK
	(2) Licorice	root	cooling	+K
	(1) Fennel	seed	cooling	=VPK
	(1) Cumin	seed	cooling	=VPK
	(1) Cinnamon	bark	heating	+P

Dose: 1 teaspoon (approx. 3 gr.) twice a day with warm water and natural sugar between meals.

Dosha	(Ratio) Herb	Part of Plant	Effect on Metabolism	Effect on Dosha
Kapha	(3) Dong Quai	root	heating	+P (mildly)
	(3) Turmeric	root	heating	=VPK
	(2) Agnus Castus	seed	heating	+P
	(2) Pennyroyal	plant	heating	+P (mildly)
	(2) Licorice	root	cooling	+K
	(1) Fennel	seed	cooling	=VPK
	(1) Cumin	seed	cooling	=VPK
	(1) Ginger	root	heating	+P

Dose: 1 teaspoon (approx. 3 gr.) twice a day with warm water and honey between meals.

Dysmenorrhea
(difficult menstruation)

The information for premenstrual cramps is also relevant here and can be applied. Table 15 gives some formulas that differ somewhat in that they address the constitution more than the ones given for just cramps (see Table 10, page 106). Dysmenorrhea is primarily a vata disorder and so all three formulas address vata to some extent to drive it from the uterus and back into the colon where it belongs.

Once more, it is the apana vayu that affects both pitta and the menstruation channel (srota). This is a case where a chronic imbalance of vata may exist. This can cause a drying or constriction of the plasma channel, which will deplete the plasma dhatu. This, in turn, will affect pitta, the blood dhatu, the blood channel, and the menstruation channel. Treatment aims to clear the apana vayu. Doses vary from 6–8 grams per day (2 X 3 gr. or 2 X 4 gr.), between meals with warm water or ginger tea for two to four months, depending on who it is and how long the problem has existed.

Table 15. Formulas for Treating Dysmenorrhea

Dosha	(Ratio) Herb	Part of Plant	Effect on Metabolism	Effect on Dosha
Vata	(3) Cramp Bark	bark	heating	+P
	(2) Angelica	root	heating	+P
	(2) Agnus Castus	seed	heating	+P
	(2) Mugwort	plant	heating	+P
	(2) Valerian	root	heating	+P
	(2) Marshmallow	root	cooling	+K
	(1) Cumin	seed	cooling	=VPK
	(1) Fennel	seed	cooling	=VPK
	(1) Ginger	root	heating	+P

Dose: 1 teaspoon (approx. 3 gr.) twice a day with warm water and honey between meals.

Table 15. Formulas for Treating Dysmenorrhea (cont.)

Pitta				
	(3) Cramp Bark	bark	heating	+P
	(2) Agnus Castus	seed	heating	+P
	(2) Pennyroyal	plant	heating	+P (mildly)
	(2) Licorice	root	cooling	+K
	(2) Valerian	root	heating	+P
	(1) Cumin	seed	cooling	=VPK
	(1) Fennel	seed	cooling	=VPK
	(1) Cinnamon	bark	heating	+P

Dose: 1 teaspoon (approx. 3 gr.) twice a day with warm water and natural sugar between meals.

Kapha				
	(3) Cramp Bark	bark	heating	+P
	(3) Angelica	root	heating	+P
	(2) Agnus Castus	seed	heating	+P
	(2) Pennyroyal	plant	heating	+P (mildly)
	(2) Valerian	root	heating	+P
	(2) Dandelion	root	cooling	+V
	(1) Fenugreek	seed	heating	+P
	(1) Cumin	seed	cooling	=VPK
	(1) Ginger	root	heating	+P

Dose: 1 teaspoon (approx. 3 gr.) twice a day with warm water and honey between meals.

Case History 6

A woman who had had dysmenorrhea (difficult periods) and menorrhagia (excess bleeding) for several years was experiencing a worsening of symptoms. She had a great deal of pain. Her liver function was very bad. She liked to drink and smoke socially. She had a pitta constitution. Both pitta and vata were imbalanced and her plasma and blood dhatus were disturbed. The two systems associated with these srotas were also disturbed, as was the menstruation srota. The apana vayu was disturbed and moving in the blood, carrying pitta ama (toxins) in the blood and menstruation srotas. I gave her the formula shown in Table 16 (see page 118). After one cycle, a good improvement had occurred. After three cycles, she felt 80 percent better. After four cycles, she was 90 percent cured. Her lifestyle was not supportive, although some dietary changes were made. Her digestion improved immediately, showing that it had been the root cause of her problems, it in turn was affected by erratic vata-type behavior and habits that disturbed her pitta constitution. This resulted in an imbalance of menstruation, as toxins moved throughout her body.

Table 16. Formula for Case History 6

Dosha	(Ratio) Herb	Part of Plant	Effect on Metabolism	Effect on Dosha
Pitta	(3) Gentian	root	cooling	+V
	(3) Barberry	root	heating	+V
	(2) Turmeric	root	heating	=VPK
	(2) Angelica	root	heating	+P
	(2) Black Cohosh	root	cooling	+V
	(2) Agnus Castus	seed	heating	+P
	(2) Licorice	root	cooling	+K
	(1) Fennel	seed	cooling	=VPK
	(1) Cumin	seed	cooling	=VPK
	(1) Ginger	root	heating	+P

Dose: 2 capsules, three times a day with water before meals.

Menorrhagia
(excess or irregular bleeding)

There are a number of causes for menorrhagia. Moreover, menorrhagia can sometimes indicate more severe problems. Care should be used in treating this problem and in deciding its root cause. Menorrhagia can result from hormonal imbalance or as a part of premenopause. It results primarily from a pitta imbalance, as it involves blood circulation and flow. Abortions, miscarriages, endometritis, and IUDs can all be causes of menorrhagia. The formulas given in Table 17 (see page 119) work to balance the endocrine system, the pitta dosha, and the constitutional type.

As pitta increases, whether from mental stress, food, or lifestyle, it moves into the blood srota. It involves the ranjaka pitta. Often, the liver/gallbladder/spleen functions have been affected prior to pitta moving into the menstruation srota. Treatment is mainly for pitta, purging the heat from the blood and intestinal tract, increasing organ function, and tonify the uterus. Although vata plays a secondary role as the principle of movement, it should be considered as well. Doses vary from 6–8 grams a day (2 X 3 gr. or 2 X 4 gr.), between meals with warm water or ginger tea for two to four months, depending on how long the problem has existed.

Table 17. Formulas for Treating Menorrhagia

Dosha	(Ratio) Herb	Part of Plant	Effect on Metabolism	Effect on Dosha
Vata	(3) Agnus Castus	seed	heating	+P
	(3) Burdock	root	cooling	+V
	(2) Angelica	root	heating	+P
	(2) Raspberry	plant	cooling	+V
	(1) Fennel	seed	cooling	=VPK
	(1) Cinnamon	bark	heating	+P
	(1) Ginger	root	heating	+P
	(¼) Saffron	flower	cooling	=VPK

Dose: 1 teaspoon (approx. 3 gr.) twice a day with warm water and honey between meals.

Dosha	(Ratio) Herb	Part of Plant	Effect on Metabolism	Effect on Dosha
Pitta	(3) Raspberry	plant	cooling	+V
	(3) Burdock	root	cooling	+V
	(2) Agnus Castus	seed	heating	+P
	(2) Yarrow	leaves	cooling	+V
	(2) Angelica	root	heating	+P
	(2) Licorice	root	cooling	+K
	(1) Fennel	seed	cooling	=VPK
	(1) Cinnamon	bark	heating	+P
	(¼) Saffron	flower	cooling	=VPK

Dose: 1 teaspoon (approx. 3 gr.) twice a day with warm water and natural sugar between meals.

Table 17. Formulas for Treating Menorrhagia (cont.)

Kapha	(3)Angelica	root	heating	+P
	(3) Burdock	root	cooling	+V
	(2) Agnus Castus	seed	heating	+P
	(2) Yarrow	leaves	cooling	+V
	(2) Dandelion	root	cooling	+V
	(1) Fenugreek	seed	heating	+P
	(1) Cumin	seed	cooling	=VPK
	(1) Ginger	root	heating	+P
	(¼) Saffron	flower	cooling	=VPK

Dose: 1 teaspoon (approx. 3 gr.) twice a day with warm water and honey between meals.

Leukorrhea
(abnormal discharge)

Any abnormal discharge is called leukorrhea. It includes any kind of yeast infection (thrush) or creamy discharge. It indicates that the internal flora have been disturbed. Normally, the vagina has a slightly acidic quality. When this is disrupted, bacteria and fungi can propagate rapidly. Discharges may be accompanied by itching and burning around the opening of the vagina.

This can be caused by tiredness, imbalance in the intestinal tract, excessive sexual intercourse, improper hygiene, or the use of "personal hygiene" products that contain perfumes or chemicals. Antibiotics are also a major cause of yeast infections. Avoid antibiotics if you have a sensitivity in this direction. Some contraceptive pills have been known to cause leukorrhea as well. Synthetic underwear and nylons can also imbalance the internal milieu of the vagina. Cotton underwear does not do this because it breathes. A poor diet, high in sugar, coffee, or alcohol, can also contribute to vaginal imbalance.

Leukorrhea is mostly a kapha disorder that involves the plasma and menstruation srotas, but it can also include the other two humors. If this is a chronic problem for you, you need a program to balance your digestive system and a change in diet. You probably have high kapha and low agni. The main focus should be on the state of agni in chronic cases. A two-week course of acidophilus capsules is needed, along with a few digestive spices like the ones used in the book: cumin, fennel, and fenugreek. Mix equal parts of the spices and grind into a powder, take ½ teaspoon before each meal for two weeks. Or you can use the formulas given in Table 18. Add ghee to the pitta formula to increase agni. Ginger powder can be used for the vata and kapha formulas to increase agni. Treatment is most effective when applied externally (as a vaginal douche). The herbal formulas are only supportive of this treatment, as they lower kapha and detoxify the digestive system, blood, and vagina. The treatments in Table 18 are given as both internal formulas and as douches.

Table 18. Formulas for Treating Leukorrhea

Dosha	(Ratio) Herb	Part of Plant	Effect on Metabolism	Effect on Dosha
Vata Internal formula	(3) Golden Seal	root	cooling	+V
	(2) Echinacea	root	cooling	+V
	(2) Barberry	root	heating	+V
	(2) Gentian	root	cooling	+V
	(1) Cardamom	seed	heating	+P
	(1) Cumin	seed	cooling	=VPK
	(1) Ginger	root	heating	+P

Dose: 2 grams three times a day with warm water and honey, one hour before eating. *Do not take this formula for longer than ten days or less than six days.*

Table 18. Formulas for Treating Leukorrhea (cont.)

Vata Douche	(1) Golden Seal	root	cooling	+V
	(1) Turmeric	root	heating	=VPK
	(1) Licorice	root	cooling	+K

Make a decoction from the roots. Use 1 cup of this body-temperature liquid twice a day as a vaginal douche.

OR

Mix ¼ cup of plain yogurt with 1 capsule of acidophilus. Apply with douche before bed, keep inside the vagina for 20–30 minutes.

Pitta Internal formula	(3) Golden Seal	root	cooling	+V
	(2) Echinacea	root	cooling	+V
	(2) Barberry	root	heating	+V
	(2) Turmeric	root	heating	=VPK
	(2) Gentian	root	cooling	+V
	(1) Cardamom	seed	heating	+P
	(1) Cumin	seed	cooling	=VPK

Dose: 2 grams three times a day with warm water and honey, one hour before eating. *Do not take this formula for longer than ten days or less than six days.*

Pitta Douche	(1) Golden Seal	root	cooling	+V
	(1) Gentian	root	cooling	+V
	(1) Turmeric	root	heating	=VPK

Make a decoction from the roots. Use 1 cup of this body-temperature liquid twice a day as a vaginal douche.

Kapha Internal formula	(3) Golden Seal	root	cooling	+V
	(2) Echinacea	root	cooling	+V
	(2) Barberry	root	heating	+V
	(1) Black Pepper	seed	heating	+P
	(1) Cardamom	seed	heating	+P
	(1) Cumin	seed	cooling	=VPK
	(1) Ginger	root	heating	+P

Dose: 2 grams three times a day with warm water and honey, one hour before eating. *Do not take this formula for longer than ten days or less than six days.*

Table 18. Formulas for Treating Leukorrhea (cont.)

Kapha Douche	(1) Golden Seal (1) Turmeric (1) Ginger	root root root	cooling heating heating	+V =VPK +P

Make a decoction from the roots. Use 1 cup of this body-temperature liquid twice a day as a vaginal douche.

Vaginitis

This is primarily a vata disturbance, which can come from the mental aggravation of vata or any chronic vata disturbance that moves into the vagina through the apana vayu and vayu srota. The formula for douches given for leukorrhea in Table 18 (see page 121–123) can be used in treatment. Internal herbs are not really needed in this condition. It is better to address diet and lifestyle to lower vata in general and to balance the digestion.

Creams are useful for treating symptoms and can be used for all constitutions. Use either marigold or calendula creams (available from your herbalist or health food store). Add 5 drops each of golden seal and chamomile tinctures for each teaspoon of cream. Mix and apply as needed.

Diet and stress are key factors in vaginitis. Often, a change in diet will bring relief from reoccurring vaginitis. If burning is involved, the bhrajaka and ranjaka pittas are involved. Purging pitta from the digestive system and rebuilding intestinal flora can be effective internal treatments. Coffee, tea, white sugar, alcohol, and smoking should be avoided to aid the healing process.

CHAPTER TEN

Premenopause

She is incarnate as Thou, and always abides in my heart.

—Tripura Rahasya

There is so much hype and misinformation around the period of time before menopause that it is hard to know what is true and what is not. This period of time is referred to as premenopause and it often begins in the late 30s or early 40s. It is a time when the body is changing. It is not a disease; it is not something to be afraid of or to ignore. Women, as a group, are trained to dread this time, because society has stigmatized it as somehow related to growing old.

One client of mine had a frightening reaction to the changes in her body. She had several problems with her body and came to me for those disturbances. Her pulse showed that her endocrine function was disturbed, among other things. She told me that she was puzzled by a strange thing: some nights she would wake up soaked with sweat, so wet that she needed to change the sheets. When I told her that, at 38, she was having premenopausal symptoms, she changed the subject!

This is a frightening situation because it means she might ignore early signs (not to mention discomfort) that could help her to seek natural support for her body. I made her a formula that would help not only her other physical problems, but cure the night sweats as well. I told her there was no need to be afraid of the changes in her body. They did not indicate anything other than a change in metabolism. In fact, all of menopause is simply that—a change in metabolic function. It is not a disease or a problem, unless proper support for the body is not given. Ayurveda can supply this support better than any one system alone, because it is so comprehensive in its therapeutic approach. Your happiness is the most important factor in all therapeutic approaches.

With the mounds of misinformation in the media and in books, it is hard to know what to believe. Here is some information that I have collected over the years about premenopause and menopause that should help to dispel certain myths.

Menopause and premenopause are not deficiencies or diseases. So the whole question of "replacement therapy" is absurd from the beginning. Menopause is a metabolic change that affects the mind and the body. It is just that, and no more—a change. Change is the one constant in life and in nature. You might even perceive "replacement therapy" as an attempt to stop life or change which, in any system, equates with death. It is more logical to assume that the *prevention* of a natural process (menopause) is disease-causing than that the process itself is a problem.

Over 50 percent of women do not experience problems in premenopause or in menopause. Only 15 percent of women who are "eligible" for hormone replacement therapy (HRT) take it. Over half of all women who have tried HRT or ERT stop within three months because of unwanted side effects. The long-term effects of HRT and ERT are not known. The side effects are not completely known, for either short- or long-term usage.

HRT is known to have the following side effects. It increases blood pressure and vaginal bleeding; it causes women to gain weight, have sore breasts, and suffer from nausea and vomiting. HRT causes bloating, uterine cramps, and headaches and depression. The frequency of cysts increases by 20 percent. The use of estrogen medications (ERT, HRT, or the pill) for five or more years increases the risk of heart attacks by 71 percent. Rates of gallbladder disease, diabetes, and lung disease all increase. ERT has been proven to have little effect on emotional swings and other subjective problems associated with premenopause and menopause.

Other known effects cited in medical studies include an increase in breast cancer and cardiovascular disease for women between the ages of 50 and 64 to over 40 percent. This number goes up to 70 percent in the 65–69 age group. There is a documented negative effect on the lipoproteins and HDL cholesterol from estroginic medications. ERT is proven to increase the rate of breast cancer by 40 percent. The longer you take either ERT or HRT, the greater your risk of having cancer or heart problems. This means that, if you begin HRT at 42, as many doctors advise, your chance of having cancer or cardiovascular disease at 52 is between 50 and 100 percent depending on the origin and focus of the study. These side effects have been documented in medical journals that I have read.

Although some companies are marketing "natural" forms of estrogen and progesterone products, you should be aware that these hormone groups do not occur in nature and therefore cannot be called natural except as they are produced by the human body. Much of the estrogen medication now taken is made from horse urine—a natural substance. However, the process of isolating the mare's estrogen changes its nature. In any case, mare estrogen is very different from human estrogen. One doctor has openly stated that there is no similarity between the two. Moreover, 33 percent of women who take this kind of product get a precancerous condition called uterine hyperplasia. Generally, it is only a matter of time before this condition becomes cancer of the uterus.

All of this information is well known in medical circles. However, things take on a new twist when you read in the newspaper that you, as a premenopausal woman (i.e., *all* women between 38 and 52), should take HRT in order to prevent heart disease. As scientific research shows exactly the opposite, one wonders at the motivation of the people who manufacture such products. All HRT and ERT products in fact carry warnings that, if any known heart or circulatory problems exist, the product is contraindicated. The logic here is interesting. A product that is contraindicated for heart problems, that is known to increase the risk of cardiovascular disease, is supposed to prevent heart attacks. This is further emphasized by the fact the FDA has not approved HRT or ERT as an effective therapy for heart attacks, because of a lack of clinical proof.

Not only do the estrogen and progesterone hormone groups begin to decline in premenopausal women, so do other hormone groups, like the glucocorticoids that are made in the adrenal glands. This group includes the now-famous DHEA and cortisone among other hormones. It is naive to think that, when taking these individual hormones, you will experience no side effects, since you are disrupting the rest of the endocrine functions of the body. This is also true for melatonin. Intelligent people should look at the many side effects attributed to the isolation of hormones from their natural environments and apply that lesson to melatonin and DHEA. Put two and two together!

The second justification used in the media and by the medical community is that taking HRT or ERT prevents osteoporosis. Yet there is no study that shows that either therapy helps the body to absorb calcium. Estrogen is proven to suppress bone-cell death. This is given as a justification for the use of ERT or HRT as a medication to prevent osteoporosis. However, if the therapy is stopped, then within a short time all benefit to the bones is lost. It is clear that, if you takes HRT for ten years to prevent the loss of calcium and then stop, within a year the benefits will be gone. But the increase in your chance of having breast or uterine cancers, or cardiovascular disease will have increased from 50 percent to over 100 percent. Is this an acceptable form of treatment for you?

Dr. Nancy Beckham wrote, in the *Australian Journal of Medical Herbalism* (volume 7(2), in 1995):

> In spite of all the known disadvantages and lack of good supportive data, women are still being pressured to take these potent hormonal drugs. If you add up all the warnings, cautions, contraindications and side effects, the number comes to over 100. The author is amazed that anyone would want to produce these drugs, let alone prescribe them.

Dr. R. Hoover published a paper in the prestigious *Elsvier Medical Journal* in Holland (1980) stating:

> Not only is the human species currently participating in a massive experiment to evaluate the potential carcinogenicity of these compounds (oestrogenic drugs), but the public health significance of even small alterations in carcinogenic risk due to these drugs is substantial.

Dr. Hoover is simply stating that the risk is enormous to society as a whole, with the full ramifications with regard to cancer and perhaps other problems unknown. Is this the image you had of modern medicine? Is this, perhaps, an indication of why over 60 percent of Americans are seeking alternative forms of medicine?

In any case, why take a chemical therapy like HRT or ERT to stop osteoporosis or heart disease in the premenopause years when statistics show these ailments are most likely to occur 20 to 30 years *after* menopause—around age 70 or 80. This logic supposes that it is better to die of cancer or heart disease at 60 than to have a fractured hip at 75. *Fifteen years of your life may be forfeit or put in danger of a serious disease simply because your body was going through a natural metabolic change.*

Osteoporosis can be prevented very easily by one scientifically proven method—eat a low protein diet. In other words, become a vegetarian. This has been common knowledge in the medical community for over twenty years. In fact, numerous studies have tried to produce a diet in which you *do not* get enough protein. These studies have all failed, except one, in which highly processed foods and "junk" foods consisting mostly of sugar were used. Vegetarian women have 25 percent fewer bone fractures between the ages of 60 and 90 than women eating high-protein diets.

Another piece of misinformation current in the media is that taking calcium supplements can prevent bone loss of calcium. In 1984, the *British Medical Journal* published a study that showed that calcium intake had no relation to bone loss of calcium. This study was substantiated by another, done at the Mayo Clinic, which showed that there was no evidence of a relationship between calcium intake and bone density. These studies have not been proven wrong in over twenty years. In fact, newer studies continue to arrive at the same conclusion—taking calcium supplements does not prevent osteoporosis.

There is, however, ample scientific evidence to show that high-protein diets—those based on animal proteins—are the primary cause of the loss of bone density. This is not an area of controversy in the medical community. High-protein diets are the main cause of osteoporosis in the United States. The most important change you can make if you want to prevent osteoporosis is to become a vegetarian, not to take HRT or calcium supplements. This, coupled with daily exercise, has been proven more effective than any other known therapy. *This approach should be started in the premenopause years, not once menopause has happened.*

Another factor in preventing osteoporosis is the elimination of the following items from your weekly diet (weekends don't count unless you are at high risk!): smoking, coffee, caffeine, white sugar, alcohol, table salt, phosphates, carbonated drinks, diuretics, and antacids that have aluminum in them. All of these steal calcium from your bones. Stop consuming them and you go a long way toward preventing bone fractures or collapse in your later years. I have read a study that showed that a vegetarian diet, a supportive lifestyle, and herbal supplements all contributed to a calcium *gain* in bones in women over 60 years of age. This study might not be accepted by many doctors or researchers, but it does indicate what Ayurveda has known for years—it is possible to rejuvenate the body.

The Ayurvedic Perspective

Illness, according to Ayurveda, is an imbalance in the three doshas or humors. What, then, is a change of metabolism? If menopause is not a deficiency disease, then what is it and how do we treat it, if at all?

Ayurveda considers premenopause to be a time where reflection is needed. The direction of your life and its ultimate goals should be questioned and reflected upon. External changes may or may not be needed. Internal changes are certain to be needed, or conflict may arise in the mind and body. These changes may be small, or they may be significant. The emphasis is best placed on your internal world—the ideas, concepts, and values that you hold. These may need to be revised and changed. You may need to open up to aspects of yourself that you had left hidden.

As you approach this time of life, your role will change if you have children. You will grow away from each other and your definition of yourself as a woman may be affected by this change. If you do not have children, you may feel a need to change your self-definition with regard to your career or society. Or all of the above. The essence of these changes is a deep primal calling from your soul. The real question is not your external environment or even your internal world—it is a question of who you are. What is your true nature? Are you limited to your temple, the body? Are you limited to your servant, the mind? Or are you some manifestation of conscious awareness that is beyond description? The time leading up to menopause and menopause itself is the time when Prakruti—Mother Nature—dives back into Purusha—pure consciousness.

This is so fundamental to a woman, yet it is completely forgotten. Women frequently wonder why men are so unintelligent (I can say this because I am a man). The answer lies in the process that I have just described. Nature forces a woman back into herself to find her real fundamental source of being. Men also are thrown back, but through the intellect, not the body, sensations, and feelings. This time is a gift and a woman who passes through it in a true sense (not just physically) becomes beautiful, wise, and nurturing in the highest sense of the words.

It is our failure as a society to understand this process that has led to the further suppression of real femininity and the destruction of the planet. The materialistic treatment of premenopause and menopause is simply a reflection of complete ignorance. To treat this opportunity as an illness is nothing short of stupid, from the Ayurvedic point of view—the deeper meaning of the process being completely negated by force.

Your first obligation is honor yourself and assist your body through this change. Follow the physical lead—the finger pointing at the moon—to dive within and find the source of all femininity, the substratum of being.

If you don't assist your body, the physical symptoms can be distracting and troublesome. If symptoms are evident, you have either been ignoring your body for some time, or you are ignoring a deeper urge. Most women in ancient India experienced no remarkable changes or symptoms. One day, they just stopped menstruating. This is still the case in many places of the world. Many progressive doctors are attributing the upsurge of premenopausal problems to the saturation of our environment and food chain with estrogenic chemicals. Others feel that women are expected to be both man and woman in today's world—strong, competitive, unfeeling, and ruthless, and then a loving mother, wife, and companion who cares for everyone—all while cleaning the house, doing the laundry, and running the car pool. Still others have documented the relation between cultural attitudes and the ease with which women pass through menopause. I feel that all factors are extremely important—not the least of which is that 60 percent of adult Americans are overweight from poor nutritional habits.

Femininity in general is suppressed and not respected by Western society, especially in the United States. Femininity today is confined to sex appeal. Models and the fashion industry are run by people who do not value a normal female body. All of these conflicts and contradictions prevent the basic needs of women from being met, thus causing difficulties in menopause and the time leading up to it.

The physical things you can do to prepare for these changes are to exercise regularly, eat a natural diet, and begin to rejuvenate your body with herbs. Many symptoms, like hot flashes, have disappeared as a result of dietary changes alone. In fact, clinical studies show that a combination of a natural diet low in protein and regular exercise are as effective as HRT. Smoking cigarettes has been shown to affect estrogen levels and contribute to hot flashes. Start with a healthy lifestyle if you are having problems. If you are not having problems, start anyway.

In Ayurveda, any signs of premenopause relate directly to the seventh tissue level, or the shukra dhatu. If there are obvious signs of deficiency, the seventh level should be nourished and rejuvenated. The most basic way to do this is through the methods given above—diet and exercise. Of course, all the other six tissues must be nourished before the food essence reaches the seventh level, so one must start with the basic treatment—diet. Then herbs can be taken to strengthen the seventh level directly. Dong quai, comfrey root, marshmallow root, licorice, ashwagandha, ginseng, and shatavari are some of my personal favorites for nourishing shukra.

The main approach in Ayurveda is one of tonics and strengthening and supporting the body. Ayurveda does not treat menopause as a disease because it is a natural part of life.

Some common signs of premenopause, from an Ayurvedic perspective are:

Irregular menstruation cycles (vata endocrine function);
Missed menstruation (vata and pitta, possible kapha block);
Missed cycle, then normal for a long time (vata endocrine function);
Depression (vata endocrine function);
Mood swings (vata endocrine function);
Sleep disturbances (vata and pitta endocrine function);
Decreased memory (all humors);
Changing sexuality (vata endocrine function);
Change of menstrual flow (heavier or lighter) (pitta endocrine function);
Hot and cold waves in the body (vata and pitta endocrine function);
Hot flashes (pitta endocrine function);
Night sweats (pitta endocrine function);
Changing skin and hair (all humors);
A small but noticeable weight gain (vata and pitta endocrine function);
Digestive changes (pitta endocrine function);
Fatigue (vata endocrine function).

I have had very good success in treating all these premenopause symptoms by using the following formulas as a base for each constitutional type. I generally get about 55 percent positive results when no dietary changes are made. When a woman changes her diet along with taking the herbal supplements, the treatment has been over 80 percent effective in eliminating all symptoms within six months. So far, in every case where a woman has changed her diet and lifestyle along with taking herbal supplements, the result has been 100 percent positive. The last category represents a minority of my clients, so further research is needed. Yet, the established trend is indeed encouraging.

Table 19 gives formulas that should be taken for a minimum of three months and for up to one year. Three to six months is an average time for 85 to 95 percent of all symptoms to disappear. Before taking these formulas, you should be sure that a heavy film (toxins) is not present on the tongue. This film should be removed by taking a detox formula or adding barberry (Berberis vulgaris) and turmeric (Curcuma longa) in a ratio of 3:2 if there is a heavy coating or 2:1 if there is a mild coating. In general, if the tongue has a coating it is best to find out why it is there—seeking the advice of a professional practitioner is advised.

Table 19. Formulas for Treating Premenopausal Symptoms

Dosha	(Ratio) Herb	Part of Plant	Effect on Metabolism	Effect on Dosha
Vata	(3) Angelica	root	heating	+P
	(2) Cramp Bark	bark	heating	+P
	(2) Black Cohosh	root	cooling	+V
	(2) Agnus Castus	seed	heating	+P
	(2) Licorice	root	cooling	+K
	(2) Nettles	plant	cooling	+V
	(1) Cumin	seed	cooling	=VPK
	(1) Fennel	seed	cooling	=VPK
	(1) Ginger	root	heating	+P

Dose: 1 teaspoon (approx. 3 gr.) twice a day with warm water and honey between meals.

Dosha	(Ratio) Herb	Part of Plant	Effect on Metabolism	Effect on Dosha
Pitta	(3) Agnus Castus	seed	heating	+P
	(2) Black Cohosh	root	cooling	+V
	(2) Angelica	root	heating	+P
	(2) Licorice	root	cooling	+K
	(2) Nettles	plant	cooling	+V
	(1) Cumin	seed	cooling	=VPK
	(1) Fennel	seed	cooling	=VPK
	(1) Cinnamon	bark	heating	+P

Dose: 1 teaspoon (approx. 3 gr.) twice a day with warm water and sugar between meals.

Table 19. Formulas for Treating Premenopausal Symptoms (cont.)

Kapha	(3) Cramp Bark	bark	heating	+P
	(3) Angelica	root	heating	+P
	(2) Agnus Castus	seed	heating	+P
	(2) Black Cohosh	root	cooling	+V
	(2) Dandelion	root	cooling	+V
	(2) Nettles	plant	cooling	+V
	(1) Fenugreek	seed	heating	+P
	(1) Cumin	seed	cooling	=VPK
	(1) Ginger	root	heating	+P

Dose: 1 teaspoon (approx. 3 gr.) twice a day with warm water and honey between meals.

Case History 7

A woman came to me with irregular menstruations, poor sleeping patterns, and general unease in the body. She was 48 and of a pitta constitution, with a vata/pitta imbalance. Pitta (fire) toxins were present on the tongue and in the body. She had some minor digestive problems and the beginning signs of malabsorption of nutrients. Vata had pushed into pitta, disturbing it and the digestive system. Her kidneys were weak due to chronic vata disturbance and the overheating nature of her pitta constitution. None of the tissue levels were deficient or damaged. Some disturbance was evident in the nerve tissue level (majja dhatu) and nerve channel (majja srota). Vata was both affected and affecting the endocrine system. I suggested 20 drops of tincture of chaste berry (Vitex agnus castus) twice a day for immediate relief, because she had an important job and was under stress at that time. This balanced endocrine function (especially progesterone). After two months, I saw her again and her menstrual problems had almost completely cleared using just the tincture, which I told her to stop for fear of possible aggravation of vata. I had also given her an herbal formula for her digestive problems, which were 80 percent cured. The formula, given in Table 20, both balanced pitta and vata in the digestive system (see page 137).

She continued this formula for four months, until her digestion was normal and the toxins were gone from the body. The use of valerian to purify the nerve channels and to lower vata were essential. I then suggested a long-term treatment of shatavari (Asparagus racemosus) and dong quai (Angelica sinensis) in equal parts of 4 grams a day for the next three to four years to rejuvenate the whole body. This approach was used to correct the long-term imbalance of vata, to lower pitta, and to nourish the seventh tissue level, shukra. One year later, her symptoms are 98 percent gone. The variable factor is the amount of stress she has in her profession. In general, she is very happy and has an increase in overall energy and vitality. In low stress times, she has no symptoms. There is little lifestyle support in this case.

Table 20. Formula for Case History 7

DOSHA	(RATIO) HERB	PART OF PLANT	EFFECT ON METABOLISM	EFFECT ON DOSHA
Pitta	(3) Barberry	root	heating	+V
	(3) Gentian	root	cooling	+V
	(2) European Madder	root	cooling	+V
	(2) Turmeric	root	heating	=VPK
	(2) Valerian	root	heating	+P
	(2) Licorice	root	cooling	+K
	(2) Marshmallow	root	cooling	+K
	(1) Fennel	seed	cooling	=VPK
	(1) Cumin	seed	cooling	=VPK

Dose: 3 grams twice a day with water and natural sugar, before breakfast and dinner.

Case History 8

A film producer came to me for several problems, including very swollen breasts before the beginning of her cycle, accompanied by a general body weight gain of seven to eight pounds. She had a general feeling of unease in her body and a feeling of overall discontent—not with her family (she was married with a 5-year-old daughter), but with unknown variables (a subjective discontent in life). She had waves of fatigue and tiredness. She had fallen ill with the flu twice that year, something unusual for her. She was 44 at the time and had a vata/kapha constitution with a vata imbalance. Her digestive organs where producing too much bile, yet her agni (ability to digest) was low. Her system was not toxic, yet the beginnings of a malabsorption syndrome were beginning in her intestinal system, contributing to her overall tiredness. The lymphatic system was congested from the disturbance of vata. This was aggravating kapha in the body, causing her to retain water. The plasma dhatu was also affected by the beginning of undernourishment to the other dhatus. With both the plasma and the lymph affected, her immune response was impaired. I suggested the formula given in Table 21 (see page 139).

I saw her a month later and she had gone through some strong emotional waves, yet her breasts were less sore before her menstruation. I saw her after two months and she felt 70 percent better, and had experienced less weight gain in her body and breasts. Her moods had stabilized, yet there was uncertainty in her professional life, which was adding stress to her life. She was extremely happy with the results and is continuing treatment for long-term support for her body. Her digestive problems, combined with a part kapha constitution, opened her up to water retention. By correcting her digestive problems and giving dandelion as a mild diuretic we were able to cut the source of the problem. Addressing the imbalanced vata with life-style therapies and herbs was the primary factor in reversing the trend, as vata was congesting kapha and causing the water retention.

In all treatments, whether for yourself or others, the digestive system must be addressed. The state of vata is also of prime concern, because it can move into either pitta or kapha, as in the two case studies above.

Table 21. Formula for Case History 8

Dosha	(Ratio) Herb	Part of Plant	Effect on Metabolism	Effect on Dosha
Vata/ Kapha	(3) Cramp Bark	bark	heating	+P
	(3) Agnus Castus	seed	heating	+P
	(3) Dandelion	root	cooling	+V
	(2) Angelica	root	heating	+P
	(2) Nettles	plant	cooling	+V
	(2) St. John's Wort	plant	cooling	+V
	(2) Turmeric	root	heating	=VPK
	(2) Gentian	root	cooling	+V
	(1) Nutmeg	nut	heating	+P
	(1) Fennel	seed	cooling	=VPK
	(1) Cumin	seed	cooling	=VPK
	(1) Ginger	root	heating	+P

Dose: 3 grams twice a day with warm water and honey before meals.

In the first study, vata was disturbing the endocrine system, the nervous system, and pitta. As the patient's constitution was pitta, this was natural and bound to happen. In the second example, vata was disturbing the endocrine system, the digestive system, and the lymphatic system, and lowering agni—the digestive ability. The failure to address vata and the digestive functions would have resulted in a partial cure or outright failure.

One very important aspect of using tonic herbs to strengthen the reproductive tissues and ojas is that *the body must be free of toxins and digesting food correctly.* Failure to follow this rule increases the toxins in your body, further lowers your immunity, and causes many kinds of disease. Hence, the rule in Ayurveda is that rejuvenating herbs (tonic herbs that build all seven tissue levels of the body) must be given only after the body is clear of all toxins and the agni is sufficient to digest the herbs.

This factor alone is a cause of failure for Western herbalists. Herbs like angelica, dong quai, licorice, marshmallow, comfrey root, shatavari, ashwagandha, bala, and ginseng must all be given when the body is clean and able to process them because they are heavy to digest.

The above herbs are my favorites for rejuvenating the body and preparing for menopause. If the above advice is followed, the results are usually excellent. I suggest the following guidelines for the use of these herbs for each constitutional type. If strong nervousness or high stress is present, add ashwagandha for one year and then remove it. Women can take ashwagandha for up to one year, but longer is not advised.

Vata: Shatavari, dong quai, and licorice. Use all plants in equal amounts. They are more effective, however, if taken in the following formula:

(3) Shatavari	(2) Bala
(3) Dong Quai	(1) Cumin
(2) Ashwagandha	(1) Fennel
(2) Licorice	(1) Ginger

Dose: 3 grams of powder twice daily with warm water (or warm whole milk) and honey between meals.

Pitta: Shatavari, licorice, marshmallow root, comfrey root, and bala. The following formula is more effective than equal amounts of the above.

(3) Shatavari	(1) Musta
(2) Licorice	(1) Cumin
(2) Marshmallow root	(1) Fennel
(1) Cinnamon	

Dose: 3 grams of powder twice daily with warm water (or whole milk), ghee, and natural sugar between meals.

Kapha: Dong quai, licorice, shatavari, ashwagandha, and ginseng. The following formula is more effective than equal amounts of the above.

(3) Dong Quai	(1) Cumin
(2) Shatavari	(1) Fenugreek
(2) Ashwagandha	(1) Ginger
(1) Licorice	

Dose: 3 grams of powder twice daily with warm water and honey between meals.

There are many other tonics, like aloe gel, but it is beyond the scope of this book to go into the many different possibilities available. The Chinese also have many other useful herbs in this regard. A study of the three herbal guides mentioned before will supply additional information where desired.

CHAPTER ELEVEN

Menopause and Postmenopause

Siva is absolute Awareness, without any form. Sri Tripura is Sakti (energy) and witness of the whole. That Being (comprising both) is perfect all round and remains undivided.

—Tripura Rahasya

Most of what was said in the previous chapter about pre-menopause applies to the time after you have stopped menstruating as well. This is a time when, for a period of ten years, you can very effectively rejuvenate your body through herbs, diet, and lifestyle. If you have started to do this in the premenopause years, or throughout your whole life, it will be even easier and more effective after menopause.

However, if you are new to natural medicine or have not followed healthy practices for other reasons, rest assured that you can start now and still have good results. Once more, I repeat that your overall health—especially that of your digestive system—is the foundation for your health as a woman.

From the time you stop menstruating, the hormones continue to change for up to ten years. It is for this reason that you can take herbs to supplement your body's needs for nutrients and the raw materials (phytosteroids) that balance endocrine functions. Sometime between 50 and 60—depending on your diet, lifestyle, and general health—you enter the vata period of life.

The positive aspects of vata are creativity, intuition, and insight. Communication and social relations are also important parts of the vata period. Deeper insights into life that result in wisdom are a very important part of the vata period. It seems that wisdom is not held in high regard by most people today. This may not actually be the case, however. Marketing forces have a hard time making money on wisdom when they can sell billions of dollars worth of products that claim to keep you young and foolish. Despite the noise of the marketplace, people may really value the wisdom that comes in the vata period of life.

Negative aspects of the vata-dominant cycle are depression, fear of death, deterioration, and anxiety. How you respond in the years after menopause—which can be half of your life if you live to be 100—depends on what you think, your daily habits, and what you ingest. If you have a positive lifestyle, attitude, and diet, you will live long, creatively, and happily. On the other hand, vata tends to go out of balance more easily as time goes on and can cause problems like arthritis, osteoporosis, and other degenerative diseases.

Your quality of life can easily be maintained or increased if you want to do so. The whole state of your life after menopause—whether it occurs naturally or by surgery—is up to you. Studies indicate that, if your life has been happy and fulfilling before menopause, it will be after it. The reverse is also true. There are few mysteries when it comes to our health. Common sense tells us that our basic attitudes in life determine our overall state of health.

A recent study, published in the April 1998 edition of the *Journal of the American Medical Association*, supported the centuries-old view of Ayurveda. The study followed 1700 people for thirty-five years and monitored their lifestyles. Those people with "good" habits and diets lived longer on the average. However, what was really striking about the conclusions of this study was that, even if the participants with "good" habits died before those with "bad" habits, they died without chronic disability. In other words, they continued to have a high-quality life right up to death, or shortly before. Therefore, the quality of your life is up to you.

As stated earlier, herbal supplements, diet, and lifestyle all are held to be equally important by the Ayurvedic system. Using the three together just makes more sense and generally delivers better results.

This has "stood up" to modern scientific studies. In a study that followed menopausal women experiencing hot flashes, diet and lifestyle were found as effective as HRT. In another study in Germany, black cohosh was found to be as effective in treating menopausal problems as ERT, with one exception—there were no side effects. Hence, we see that science has again and again found that many natural things —such as lifestyle, diet, and herbal supplements—can be as effective as invasive chemical therapies.

It should be clear to all that herbs, diet, and lifestyle cannot be patented under a brand name and marketed. This is especially true in the realm of herbal research. Who is willing to spend several million dollars on researching an herb in its totality when they will never be able to make money from the results of their findings? Obviously, our whole society would need to shift dramatically for this to become a reality. Until then, we have the ancient system and advice of Ayurveda to guide us, as it has done since the beginning of time.

One aspect of menopause, according to Ayurveda, is the need for a woman to re-evaluate her life on all levels, especially on issues of identity. If your identity is limited to your body and looking young, you will have a difficult time as the body matures and diverges from a socially desirable image. If your identity is limited to your family, this also will be changing as your children grow up and begin to live their own lives.

In the professional world, people begin to look at you only as person and not as a woman. You may feel strange and slightly disturbed by this change. Your whole professional life may become a source of questioning for you, and you may experience some dissatisfaction one way or another. It may be time to re-evaluate your profession and see how you can move into a more creative, fulfilling role in your work.

Fundamental to all of these feelings and reflections, however, is your basic identity—who you take yourself to be. This is the reason why women enter menopause, according to the ancient wisdom. It provides a period of time when a woman is confronted with herself. This causes her to question her true identity—body, mind, or soul. The ancient wisdom taught that woman (and, believe it or not, men, too!) is not limited to either of these three (body, mind, or soul). It is the discovery of the substratum of these three that is the ultimate goal and mystery of life. Your ability to penetrate this mystery is the real purpose of the body's change. It forces you inward to discover reality.

Men are not as lucky because they are not forced by physical changes. However, they also have a "menopause" that affects their mental view of the world and their perception of themselves. Many men experience a midlife crisis that is nature's way of demanding that they turn inward and find their own true identity. The question for both women and men is not the "attainment" of any goal, but the act of turning inward and questioning the nature of reality itself.

If this period of time is used constructively, it is very rewarding. Unfortunately, there is often little social or private support for women to do this. In this case, it is best to join with other women, so that a support group can provide the understanding that your partner and society should be providing.

Menopause can be a great change in how you perceive life and how you begin to interact with it. Many women are able to do this naturally. We seldom hear of these women, however, because they don't make news or sell products. Life is feminine in nature and it is calling to you during these years. Listen to it; follow it. It will lead you to happiness and wisdom.

Ayurveda treats menopause by supporting the body with nourishing herbs and foods, a supportive lifestyle, mild exercise, and inner reflection. This offers a balanced approach to the second half of your life. As mentioned before, the first five to ten years after you stop menstruating will still be a time of adjustment for your body. During this time, it is good to support the endocrine system with friendly hormone-supporting herbs. After about 60 years of age, the supplements are primarily just for strengthening and nourishing and, as always, for balancing vata as it increases with age.

The best treatment is food. A diet low in (or without) animal proteins will be the best support for your heart and bones. While it is possible to take calcium supplements (which are shown to have no effect in building calcium in the bones) and to eat calcium-rich foods and herbs, the best treatment is to stop eating high amounts of protein that rob the body of calcium faster than any other factor in life.

Ayurveda takes an additional step. The kala (membrane that separates the dhatu from the srota—i.e., the tissue from the system) is the responsible factor in calcium absorption. The kala for the bones is the colon. If you have a colon that is clogged and coated with the decayed food matter of a lifetime, your absorption of calcium (and all other nutrients) will be severely limited or impaired. This is another reason why Ayurveda stresses the health of the intestinal system as a whole.

The best general product to maintain the colon, rejuvenate it, and keep the natural elimination of waste transpiring normally is called triphala. This is a famous product that is used in every traditional household in India. It is made from three (tri) fruits (phala). Each fruit balances one of the doshas. Therefore, this product is called tri-doshic, or good for all kinds of constitutions. It has so many properties that it would require a book of pharmaceutical actions all by itself.

Some of its properties show it to effectively inhibit the HIV—as well as other—viruses, prevent aging with its antioxidant properties, rejuvenate tissues and cells, prevent cancer, increase absorption of B vitamins and other nutrients, eliminate heavy metals from the tissues, promote weight loss, regulate blood-cell production, balance digestive function, and help regulate daily elimination.[1] Triphala is not a strong laxative. It has very mild laxative effects that are stronger in pitta-type women, medium in kapha types, and almost ineffective for vata types. If you have chronic constipation, triphala alone will generally not resolve your problem.

Triphala should be used as an overall tonic and to increase the absorption of nutrients and of other herbal formulas. Triphala is included in small amounts in almost every herbal preparation in traditional Ayurvedic pharmacology. As it is not available in all parts of the United States, I have used cumin, fennel, fenugreek, ginger, and cinnamon to act as digestive stimulants throughout the formulas in this book. Triphala can be added in small amounts to any formula in this book to add the above qualities. The use of this formula in small amounts (1 gram per day) will have very beneficial effects over the years. Higher doses can be taken for other problems as well.

The two main reasons for you to take HRT and ERT (heart disease and osteoporosis) have been discussed earlier and seen to have little or no justification when benefits are compared to the dangers. Dietary changes alone are enough to prevent these problems. These beneficial effects are enhanced when the daily use of the triphala formula is added to a balanced, low-protein diet.

The main herbs that can be used in menopause and postmenopause are: dong quai, shatavari, ashwagandha, saffron, bala, aloe gel, ginseng, and formulas like Chavan Prash or other Rasayanas. I suggest you use these herbs in the following manner for each constitution:

---

[1] Atreya, *Practical Ayurveda* (York Beach, ME; Samuel Weiser, 1998), chapter 8.

Vata

(3) Shatavari	(1) Cumin
(3) Dong Quai	(1) Fennel
(2) Ashwagandha	(1) Ginger
(2) Licorice	

Dose: 3 grams of powder twice daily with warm water (or whole milk) and honey between meals.

Pitta

(3) Shatavari	(1) Fennel
(2) Licorice	(1) Cinnamon
(2) Dong Quai	(¼) Saffron
(1) Cumin	

Dose: 3 grams of powder twice daily with warm water (or whole milk), ghee, and natural sugar between meals.

Kapha

(3) Dong Quai	(1) Cumin
(2) Ashwagandha	(1) Fenugreek
(2) Shatavari	(1) Ginger

Dose: 3 grams of powder twice daily with warm water and honey between meals.

Case History 9

A woman came to see me on the advice of her sister. She was 59 and had suffered from strong hot flashes, night sweats, and heat waves for the last six years. She had found some relief in homeopathy and vitamin supplements, but was not really satisfied with the results. The sweats had tapered off substantially, but were still occasionally present. The patient was a pitta/vata type with a vata imbalance. Pitta was also slightly imbalanced, because vata was pushing into it. She had pitta toxins in the digestive tract but was in generally good health. She complained of feeling bloated and puffy, which was the primary reason she came to me. Her water metabolism was imbalanced and she had weak kidney function. She lived a very social life and enjoyed eating and drinking. Her sleep habits were regular, but not in keeping with the day (3am to 10am)! Therefore, she was giving her body little life-style support, other than eating and drinking high-quality food and wine. I suggested the formulas shown in Table 22.

Table 22. Formula 1 for Case History 9

DOSHA	(RATIO) HERB	PART OF PLANT	EFFECT ON METABOLISM	EFFECT ON DOSHA
Pitta/ Vata	(3) Uva Ursi	plant	cooling	+V
	(2) Cramp Bark	bark	heating	+P
	(2) Agnus Castus	seed	heating	+P
	(2) Angelica	root	heating	+P
	(2) Licorice	root	cooling	+K
	(2) Valerian	root	heating	+P
	(1) Calamus*	root	heating	+P
Dose: 3 grams twice a day with warm water and natural sugar.				

*Internal use is currently restricted by the FDA in the United States.

The first formula supported her endocrine function and water metabolism, and brought vata into balance. When I saw her four months later, she was no longer bloated and the other symptoms where 75 percent better. I also gave her a liver-cleansing formula to take at the same time (see Table 23, page 151) she took the liver formula for three months. When she finished the above formula, I changed her formula to the following because she still had toxins present in the digestive tract, even though liver function had improved. Vata had come down significantly and was balanced. She took this formula for another three months and then stopped taking any herbs because her symptoms were 95 percent gone. She continued to take vitamin supplements. She also complained of having good digestion after the treatment.

Table 23. Formula 2 for Case History 9

Dosha	(Ratio) Herb	Part of Plant	Effect on Metabolism	Effect on Dosha
Pitta/ Vata	(2) Uva Ursi	plant	cooling	+V
	(2) Barberry`	root	heating	+V
	(2) Turmeric	root	heating	=VPK
	(2) Angelica	root	heating	+P
	(2) Licorice	root	cooling	+K
	(1) Calamus *	root	heating	+P
	(1) Fennel	seed	cooling	=VPK

Dose: 3 grams twice a day with warm water and natural sugar.

*Internal use is currently restricted by the FDA in the United States.

Case History 10

A woman 48 years old came to see me. She had stopped menstruating one year before and was suffering from many small symptoms of menopause—heat waves, sweating at night, mood swings, generally feeling strangely with no energy. She had suffered from food allergies for many years and ate a mostly vegetarian diet. She was a professional woman and traveled a lot for her work. She was pitta, with a chronic imbalance of vata (as seen in food sensitivities). She had pitta toxins present and her whole metabolism was out of balance. Her agni was low and she took lots of vitamins and minerals (which is one reason why her agni was low). Her kidneys were weak and her water metabolism was deranged. I suggested that she take the formula given in Table 24 (see page 152) for three months.

Table 24. Formula for Case History 10

Dosha	(Ratio) Herb	Part of Plant	Effect on Metabolism	Effect on Dosha
Pitta	(3) Licorice	root	cooling	+K
	(3) Agnus Castus	seed	heating	+P
	(3) Angelica	root	heating	+P
	(2) Gentian	root	cooling	+V
	(2) Turmeric	root	heating	=VPK
	(1) Barberry	root	heating	+V
	(1) Uva Ursi	plant	cooling	+V
	(1) Fennel	seed	cooling	=VPK
	(1) Cumin	seed	cooling	=VPK
	(1) Fenugreek	seed	heating	+P
Dose: 3 grams twice a day with warm water.				

The patient avoided all sweets and took the powder naturally. I also suggested that she take 4 grams of shatavari every day for a year. She felt much better emotionally in three months and was almost completely free from the symptoms of menopause. Her digestive problems took a few months longer to clear and she still has some food sensitivity, mostly due to the high-vata lifestyle. The shatavari will continue to nourish her reproductive system and her kidneys.

Vaginal Dryness

Another problem that menopausal and postmenopausal women face is a dry vagina. This is due to high vata, especially apana vayu. The treatment should first concentrate on lowering vata in the constitution and then on supplementing the reproductive organs with the long-term use of shatavari. I suggest 4 to 8 grams of Shatavari a day. I have had mixed success with this approach, as it depends on how much the woman is willing to change vata habits and lifestyle. Shatavari has the advantage of being a demulcent herb (one that nourishes and lubricates), as well as a good hormone supplement.

Demulcent herbs, such as marshmallow and licorice, taken as decocted teas are sometimes enough. For other women, the tea and sesame oil should be mixed together and used internally as a douche (allowing it to stay for as long as possible—up to 30 minutes—before intercourse), while still drinking the tea. If none of these works, I recommend sesame oil alone as a douche before intercourse. Use only the cold-pressed natural sesame oil that you can buy in a health food store. Do not use the cooked oriental variety of oil commonly available, as it has no medicinal value.

One reoccurring theme that I noticed in my files as I reviewed them for this book was that, invariably, some digestive problems accompany hormone imbalance. I personally draw the conclusion, after looking back over several hundred cases, that one cannot separate the overall metabolic function from the endocrine system. The more I use the Ayurvedic methodology of balancing constitution and humors, the better the results I get and the better my clients feel.

CHAPTER TWELVE

Cysts, Fibroids, and Tumors

When the Supreme Goddess is well pleased with the worship of the devotee, She turns into vichara (discrimination, investigation) in him and shines as the blazing Sun in the expanse of his heart.

—Tripura Rahasya

It is now estimated that 20–40 percent of all women will have fibroids at least once in their life. Fibroids are now so common that they are considered "normal" in the United States. Ayurveda perceives this situation as far from normal. One of the primary causes of this phenomenon, according to many modern doctors, is the dramatic increase of estrogenic chemicals in the food chain. Devitalized diets and junk foods also play a major role. Hence, Ayurvedic therapies are extremely effective in eliminating fibroids, cysts, and benign tumors.

The modern medical community has treated the increase of fibroids with surgery—until recently, only hysterectomies. This is the most invasive treatment possible for a problem that can be resolved with diet, lifestyle, and herbs. The question here is what are you willing to do? Are you willing to put some time and energy into healing yourself or are you willing to be just a hunk of meat on the operating table? If you feel this to be a strong image, I suggest you talk to people who have had this or other kinds of surgery. There are compassionate, humane doctors. Unfortunately, the ones that usually have to function within the context of a hospital or clinic are seldom humane or compassionate due to stress and workload.

If you are willing to take responsibility for your health—and perhaps the whole creative aspect of your life—you can heal yourself. There are exceptions to this. I am not saying that Ayurveda cures all disease all the time. It is simply my experience that every woman who has come to me with either a cyst or fibroids has been cured through her own efforts and Ayurveda. So the real question here is: What are you willing to do to get well?

Ayurveda perceives this category of problems as an accumulation of kapha in the body. This can happen for two primary reasons: an overproduction of the kapha humor in the body and constricted vata, which also causes congestion. Both of these situations can cause a blockage or congestive situation in the plasma dhatu and the plasma srota. As discussed in chapter 3, this tissue level and system also control the lymphatic system—the site of many cysts and tumors.

When the uterus is involved, the menstruation srota is involved.[1] When the breasts are involved, the lactation srota is involved. Both of these systems are affected by the congestion of kapha in the plasma and lymph systems. Treatment depends on which system is involved and on the constitution of the woman.

In general, kapha women or kapha dual-type women are the most prone to cysts and tumors. Pitta types are more prone to have fibroids. Yet I have had several women of a pitta nature with cysts as well. It is interesting to note that, at least in one case, the woman had strong relationship problems with her mother. The link of the humors to the mind and emotions is important in the treatment of all diseases, but perhaps more so in this type of problem.

As kapha is prone to hold and accumulate emotions, it provides a prime environment for the creation of internal growths. Kapha mixes or types are also very sentimental and so may tend to feel unloved or feel a lack of love. These

---

[1] This also means that pitta is involved. Uterine fibroids primarily indicate a pitta problem, and secondarily a Kapha unbalance.

emotions can lead to a congestion of vata or life-force energy. This congestion blocks the already slow movement of kapha, causing accumulation in the tissues, dhatus.

It should be clearly understood that vata is the principle in the body (and nature) that moves things. Both pitta and kapha are immobile without vata. If vata becomes constricted, it, in turn, stops both kapha and pitta from functioning properly. When vata stops completely, death results. A vata person can have all the symptoms of a kapha person if the pranic system—the vayu srota or nadis—becomes congested or blocked. This relates primarily to the vyana and apana vayus of vata, yet other forms of vata can be involved also.

In general, there are several factors to be considered in all three of these situations: first the constitution, then the state of vata, and last the toxic state of the body. Still deeper is the function of the digestive system and, most especially, the state of agni—the digestive ability. Agni lives in the small intestine and is closely related to pitta. There are many sub-agnis that are responsible for the digestion of matter and emotions on every level of the body and mind. One of the most important of these for this discussion is that of the five liver agnis and the ranjaka pitta. These help to eliminate excess estrogens in the blood and fat. They also process many B vitamins and maintain mineral balance. If your liver and agni are not working well, you risk the problems discussed in this chapter.

Remember that the liver (pitta) relates to the menstrual flow, and that pitta controls the menstruation system directly. Hence, any problems related to pitta, agni, the liver, or the digestion in general will open you up for trouble. It is best to keep these functions working correctly, so that problems do not occur. If they do occur, you must correct these functions immediately.

Therefore, the main treatment approach in Ayurveda involves an understanding of the constitution of the person and an understanding of the vikruti, or imbalanced state. In these cases, both vata and kapha will be involved to some extent and both need to be treated accordingly. Pitta will need to addressed as well if the digestion is disturbed. Last, but never least, remember agni, the principle of fire that lives inside, transforming everything that comes into the body—food, emotions, or sensations.

Cysts

There are four basic kinds of cysts. Three are difficult to treat and require professional attention, according to your situation and health. The other, most common, kind of cyst relates to ovulation and is formed from either the FSH or LH hormones. These are called "functional" cysts and are easy to treat yourself. There are two kinds of these cysts. Because they are caused by the hormones that control ovulation, they are named Follicle (from FSH) or Luteal (from LH) cysts. Functional cysts are again considered "normal" and usually go away in two to three cycles.

Birth control pills are used by some doctors to stop ovulation in order to give the body a chance to dissolve the cysts "naturally." This ignores the fact that the endocrine function must already have been imbalanced for the cyst to form in the first place. Moreover, weak or low doses of birth control pills can cause cysts, because they are not able to sufficiently inhibit the pituitary gland. This line of treatment is symptomatic, and using the pill imbalances vata the longer you take it.

The best treatment for cysts is to balance the doshas—your constitution—and then balance the endocrine function. This has proven again and again to be the most effective treatment in naturopathic clinical trials. Balancing the endocrine function is done by balancing vata and using hormone-supporting herbs. Once more, I wish to point out that the use of many hormone-supporting herbs alone is not sufficient, as many of them imbalance vata over the long term, especially in tincture form. This can lead to other kinds of imbalances in the body, or reoccurrence of the same problem later on.

Lifestyle is very important in all treatments, and especially so for cysts, fibroids, and tumors. One of the best treatments is to have daily massage to stimulate or drain the lymphatic system. You can give yourself massage as well. This is a whole science in Ayurveda and is considered to be the prime treatment of vata. Consequently, massage is very important in the treatment of the problems discussed so far in this book. I have explained this system in *The Secrets of Ayurvedic Massage*.[2]

Massage stimulates the fat and muscle tissues which help to pacify the vata, move the kapha, and eliminate toxins lodged in the plasma and blood. It is a an important form of treatment for all ten constitutional types and most diseases. The subject is vast and Western massage is largely concerned only with techniques and structure. Ayurvedic massage is concerned with the whole metabolic function of the body, including the balance of the three humors. As such, it is much more effective, in a medical sense, than Western massage, which is often more advanced in physical techniques. Any massage will help in the elimination of toxins.

Exercise is important, because it stimulates the body and helps eliminate toxins and move kapha. Hard, aerobic types of exercise are not really beneficial from the Ayurvedic point of view, because they aggravate vata over the long term. Very strenuous activities strain vata. These kinds of sports also reduce body fat in women, which can lead to other problems—most noticeably, a reduction in estrogen and prostaglandin production. The deficiency of either of these can lead to menstrual problems and premenopausal symptoms, and perhaps speed up the aging process. A certain amount of body fat is needed for health. Lighter forms of exercise, like yoga asana, walking, dance, or lobbying your congressperson, are more beneficial in the long run than extreme or strenuous activities.

Diet should consist of lowering kapha. This means foods should be consumed that are the opposite in quality to

---

[2] Atreya, *The Secrets of Ayurvedic Massage* (Twin Lakes, WI: Lotus Press, 1999).

kapha—not creamy, rich, heavy to digest, high in protein, or cold and sticky. A diet that balances or reduces kapha consists mainly of vegetables and whole grains, with little or no meat or dairy products. Amadea Morningstar has written a few good cookbooks that give a lot of information on constructing a healing diet for Westerners using Western food.[3] Dr. Vasant Lad has also written an excellent book on self-healing with food.[4] These books can be consulted for in-depth information on these subjects. Chapter 14 gives an introduction to these ideas as well.

Promoting elimination is a primary concern. Massage and diet are the focus of this action; however we can also use herbs. Probably the best herbal preparation overall for elimination, strengthening the body, and promoting metabolic function is the triphala formula spoken of in chapter 11. The reduction and/or elimination of ama (toxins) is high on the list of treatment priorities.

Either a mild laxative like triphala or other detoxifing herbs can be used in the formula to drive ama out of the body. Many times, it is the congestion of kapha, in combination with ama, that creates the more difficult kind of cysts. Ayurveda says that accumulation of ama is behind most diseases. In this category of problems, ama is certain to be present to some extent. You can treat it by cleaning out your body and then supporting your body with a lighter diet and exercise.

Externally, castor-oil packs can be used to drive out the toxins and break up accumulations of kapha. It should be noted that castor oil has a long history of use in Ayurveda, both internally and externally. The external application with heat is very effective in stopping pain and the congestion of kapha. It also has a calming effect on vata. Castor-oil packs

---

[3] Amadea Morningstar, *Ayurvedic Cooking for Westerners* (Twin Lakes, WI: Lotus Press, 1994); and *The Ayurvedic Cookbook* (Twin Lakes, WI: Lotus Press, 1990).

[4] Vasant Lad, and Usha Lad, *Ayurvedic Cooking for Self-Healing* (Twin Lakes, WI: Lotus Press, 1994).

on the abdomen are very effective in balancing the apana vayu—the main disease-causing force in the body. For any serious uterine problem stemming from congestion, castor-oil packs are highly recommended.

Soak cotton fabric in warm castor oil. It should be wet, but not dripping wet. Lay it on the part of the body you want to treat. Cover the poultice with plastic cloth or wrap. Cover this with a towel. Over this, put a hot water bottle or heating pad on medium-low heat. Cover all of this with another towel. The idea is to have the warm oil on your body, and not all over everything else! The plastic helps to keep the oil where it should be and the heat helps to drive the already-warm oil deeper into the tissues.

Herbs that are helpful in doing away with cysts are dandelion, barberry, turmeric, wild yam, golden seal, ginger, yellow dock, guggulu, myrrh, raspberry, and chaparral. I suggest the formulas in Tables 25 and 26 (see pages 161–164) for the treatment of all forms of cysts, not only functional cysts. The formulas should be accompanied by the above supportive therapies.

Table 25. Formulas for Treating Uterine Cysts

Dosha	(Ratio) Herb	Part of Plant	Effect on Metabolism	Effect on Dosha
Vata	(3) Angelica	root	heating	+P
	(3) Barberry	root	heating	+V
	(3) Dandelion	root	cooling	+V
	(2) Black Cohosh	root	cooling	+V
	(2) Agnus Castus	seed	heating	+P
	(2) Turmeric	root	heating	=VPK
	(2) Myrrh	resin	heating	+P
	(1) Yellow Dock	root	cooling	+V
	(1) Fenugreek	seed	heating	+P
	(1) Cumin	seed	cooling	=VPK
	(1) Ginger	root	heating	+P

Dose: 1 teaspoon (approx. 3 gr.) twice a day with warm water and honey between meals.

Table 25. Formulas for Treating Uterine Cysts (cont.)

Pitta				
	(3) Barberry	root	heating	+V
	(2) Turmeric	root	heating	=VPK
	(2) Gentian	root	cooling	+V
	(2) Black Cohosh	root	cooling	+V
	(2) Agnus Castus	seed	heating	+P
	(2) Yellow Dock	root	cooling	+V
	(2) Dandelion	root	cooling	+V
	(2) Myrrh	resin	heating	+P
	(1) Cumin	seed	cooling	=VPK
	(1) Fennel	seed	cooling	=VPK
	(1) Cinnamon	bark	heating	+P

Dose: 1 teaspoon (approx. 3 gr.) twice a day with warm water and sugar between meals.

Kapha				
	(3) Angelica	root	heating	+P
	(3) Barberry	root	heating	+V
	(3) Dandelion	root	cooling	+V
	(2) Black Cohosh	root	cooling	+V
	(2) Agnus Castus	seed	heating	+P
	(2) Turmeric	root	heating	=VPK
	(2) Myrrh	resin	heating	+P
	(2) Golden Seal	root	cooling	+V
	(2) Yellow Dock	root	cooling	+V
	(1) Fenugreek	seed	heating	+P
	(1) Cumin	seed	cooling	=VPK
	(1) Ginger	root	heating	+P

Dose: 1 teaspoon (approx. 3 gr.) twice a day with warm water and honey between meals.

ATTENTION: Do not take these formulas longer than three months as they are reducing formulas, not tonics or strengthening formulas.

Table 26. Formulas for Treating Breast and Lymphatic Cysts (cont.)

DOSHA	(RATIO) HERB	PART OF PLANT	EFFECT ON METABOLISM	EFFECT ON DOSHA
Vata	(3) Barberry	root	heating	+V
	(3) Myrrh	resin	heating	+P
	(3) Dandelion	root	cooling	+V
	(2) Black Cohosh	root	cooling	+V
	(2) Agnus Castus	seed	heating	+P
	(2) Turmeric	root	heating	=VPK
	(2) Valerian	root	heating	+P
	(1) Calamus*	root	heating	+P
	(1) Yellow Dock	root	cooling	+V
	(1) Fenugreek	seed	heating	+P
	(1) Cumin	seed	cooling	=VPK
	(1) Ginger	root	heating	+P

Dose: 1 teaspoon (approx. 3 gr.) twice a day with warm water and honey between meals.

DOSHA	(RATIO) HERB	PART OF PLANT	EFFECT ON METABOLISM	EFFECT ON DOSHA
Pitta	(3) Barberry	root	heating	+V
	(3) Turmeric	root	heating	=VPK
	(2) Gentian	root	cooling	+V
	(2) Black Cohosh	root	cooling	+V
	(2) Agnus Castus	seed	heating	+P
	(2) Echinacea	root	cooling	+V
	(2) Yellow Dock	root	cooling	+V
	(2) Dandelion	root	cooling	+V
	(2) Myrrh	resin	heating	+P
	(1) Cumin	seed	cooling	=VPK
	(1) Fennel	seed	cooling	=VPK
	(1) Cinnamon	bark	heating	+P

Dose: 1 teaspoon (approx. 3 gr.) twice a day with warm water and natural sugar between meals.

* Internal use is currently resrticted by the FDA in the United States.

Table 26. Formulas for Treating Breast and Lymphatic Cysts (cont.)

Kapha	(3) Myrrh	resin	heating	+P
	(3) Barberry	root	heating	+V
	(3) Dandelion	root	cooling	+V
	(2) Turmeric	root	heating	=VPK
	(2) Black Cohosh	root	cooling	+V
	(2) Agnus Castus	seed	heating	+P
	(2) Echinacea	root	cooling	+V
	(2) Yellow Dock	root	cooling	+V
	(1) Fenugreek	seed	heating	+P
	(1) Cumin	seed	cooling	=VPK
	(1) Ginger	root	heating	+P
	(1) Black Pepper	seed	heating	+P

Dose: 1 teaspoon (approx. 3 gr.) twice a day with warm water and honey between meals.

ATTENTION: Do not take these formulas longer than three months as they are reducing formulas, not tonics or strengthening formulas. Also, the use of myrrh can be hard on the kidneys. If you have weak kidneys, monitor your state carefully. These formulas are balanced with dandelion to prevent kidney problems, yet you should be careful with the use of myrrh if you have a history of kidney problems.

Case History 11

This is an interesting case because it shows what can be done *after* a problem has come to a crisis point and the environment is perfect to create the same problem again. In many respects, this case makes it easy to understand the cause of the problem. A young woman, age 27, came to me two months after having one liter of blood drained from her pelvic cavity after a blood-filled cyst had burst. She had a pitta/kapha constitution, with an imbalance of vata and pitta. She had no indication that the cyst was there, other than some pain on urination or defication. She had been having irregular menstruations for many months, sometimes even missing a cycle completely. She was in great turmoil emotionally, because she was leaving her boyfriend of eleven years. She felt that he did not love her any more and they were drifting apart. When she came to me, her whole body was out of balance, along with her endocrine function. No treatment was given to her, other than a small incision to drain the blood out of the pelvic cavity.

She was feeling quite badly and needed emotional support, which I gave. She had no energy and generally felt poorly, yet the feeling was subjective, as there was no "disease." She complained of small digestive problems. I started treatment by giving life-style counseling, including dietary changes and encouraging her to change her personal life, as difficult as that was. She was suffering from weak kidney function, malabsorption of nutrients, and a chronic imbalance of vata. I suggested the formula given in Table 27. I saw, through diagnosis, that there still remained an amount of blood in the abdomen and pelvic cavity. The kalas were not functioning and the plasma and blood dhatus were severely affected. The two srotas controlling these dhatus were also not functioning correctly. She was in a perfect situation to create more internal cysts.

Table 27. Formula for Case History 11

DOSHA	(RATIO) HERB	PART OF PLANT	EFFECT ON METABOLISM	EFFECT ON DOSHA
Pitta/ Kapha	(3) Agnus Castus	seed	heating	+P
	(3) Turmeric	root	heating	=VPK
	(2) Black Haw	bark	heating	+P
	(2) Barberry	root	heating	+V
	(2) Gentian	root	cooling	+V
	(2) Dandelion	root	cooling	+V
	(2) Elecampane	root	heating	+P
	(2) Licorice	root	cooling	+K
	(1) Nutmeg	nut	heating	+P
	(1) Cumin	seed	cooling	=VPK
	(1) Fennel	seed	cooling	=VPK
	(1) Ginger	root	heating	+P

Dose: 3 grams twice a day with water and natural sugar before meals for ten weeks

When we met again, the patient had had one menstruation and was now late by almost four weeks for the second. I gave her a tea to bring on menstruation [(3) Mugwort and (2) Pennyroyal] which worked well. She felt very well mentally and physically was better. Her metabolic state was 100 percent improved. There were no signs of doshic or metabolic imbalance. Her endocrine function was still disturbed, but her personal life was turning around and she had a new boyfriend. The endocrine function became normal after another four months of treatment.

Fibroids

One in every four women between 30 and 50 has had, or will have, fibroids at one time in her life, according to modern studies. These facts can be changed by following an Ayurvedic program to balance your individual constitution. If you do not know how to—or are not willing to—make the effort to balance your metabolism, then these figures are very significant.

The leading cause of hysterectomies in the United States is fibroids. Three out of ten hysterectomies are performed because of fibroids. That number was over 175,000 in 1993. As mentioned at the beginning of this chapter, the primary treatment for fibroids, until recently, has been a complete hysterectomy. Fibroids are known to increase with increased estrogen and decrease with an increase of progesterone. There is an obvious relation to endocrine function and external factors, such as estrogenic chemicals in the food chain.

There are four classifications of fibroids. Nevertheless, all four types can be treated through the same Ayurvedic formulas and therapies. Each of the four can cause different problems. Some cause extreme pain when in a progressive state. Recognize the signs and prevent them from occurring in the first place.

Some of the many problems associated with fibroids are: excessive bleeding, fatigue, pelvic pain, spotting, pressure in the pelvis, lower-back pain, frequent urination, constipation, and a distortion of the uterus. All of these problems are associated with the vata dosha and primarily with the apana vayu. Fibroids, according to Ayurveda, are a constriction of the apana vayu, which causes accumulation of kapha or pitta in the pelvic area.

Balancing vata—especially the apana vayu—is the most important factor in treatment, after understanding the natal constitution. The emotional nature of vata must be understood. Vata controls the pituitary gland (the brain of the endocrine system) and is imbalanced by stress, anxiety, fear, and chronic depression. Hence, the first place to look is to see if you are happy and not holding in your feelings. Are you able to express yourself and your creativity?

Perhaps the next most important factor is to eliminate all processed and manufactured foods from your diet. This includes all forms of premade drinks (with the exception of a good Bordeaux now and then—organic of course!). Dairy products are well thought of in Ayurveda, but a different kind of dairy than what is commercially available today in the United States. All dairy products today are laced with estrogenic hormones and are therefore contraindicated for fibroids and cancers. All meats are also contraindicated, for the same reasons. These products in themselves are not necessarily thoroughly bad. However, the way they are manufactured and produced makes them detrimental to your health if you have fibroids. They should be strictly avoided if your problem is serious or if you have a reoccurring problem.

A vegetarian diet that balances kapha is the right approach, according to Ayurveda. Low protein intake will also help. Don't eat tons of tofu with the idea that you need to "make up" some "lost" protein. These ideas are not based in fact, but are rather the creation of the meat and dairy industry. Ayurveda is not against meat and dairy in and of themselves. It does understand, however, that the manner in which they are prepared can unbalance the body. Table 28 gives formulas for the reduction and removal of uterine fibroids.

Table 28. Formulas for Treating Uterine Fibroids

Dosha	(Ratio) Herb	Part of Plant	Effect on Metabolism	Effect on Dosha
Vata	(3) Black Cohosh	root	cooling	+V
	(3) Agnus Castus	seed	heating	+P
	(3) St. John's Wort	plant	cooling	+V
	(2) Wild Yam	root	cooling	=VPK
	(2) Barberry	root	heating	+V
	(2) Turmeric	root	heating	=VPK
	(2) Myrrh	resin	heating	+P
	(2) Valerian	root	heating	+P
	(1) Calamus*	root	heating	+P
	(1) Fenugreek	seed	heating	+P
	(1) Cumin	seed	cooling	=VPK
	(1) Ginger	root	heating	+P

Dose: 1 teaspoon (approx. 3 gr.) twice a day with warm water and honey between meals.

Dosha	(Ratio) Herb	Part of Plant	Effect on Metabolism	Effect on Dosha
Pitta	(3) Agnus Castus	seed	heating	+P
	(3) St. John's Wort	plant	cooling	+V
	(2) Black Cohosh	root	cooling	+V
	(2) Wild Yam	root	cooling	=VPK
	(2) Yellow Dock	root	cooling	+V
	(2) Barberry	root	heating	+V
	(2) Turmeric	root	heating	=VPK
	(2) Gentian	root	cooling	+V
	(1) Cumin	seed	cooling	=VPK
	(1) Fennel	seed	cooling	=VPK
	(1) Cinnamon	bark	heating	+P
	(¼) Saffron	flower	cooling	=VPK

Dose: 1 teaspoon (approx. 3 gr.) twice a day with warm water and natural sugar between meals.

Table 28. Formulas for Treating Uterine Fibroids (cont.)

Kapha	(3) Agnus Castus	seed	heating	+P
	(3) Myrrh	resin	heating	+P
	(2) Black Cohosh	root	cooling	+V
	(2) Wild Yam	root	cooling	=VPK
	(2) Barberry	root	heating	+V
	(2) Dandelion	root	cooling	+V
	(2) Turmeric	root	heating	=VPK
	(1) Fenugreek	seed	heating	+P
	(1) Cumin	seed	cooling	=VPK
	(1) Ginger	root	heating	+P
	(1) Black Pepper	seed	heating	+P

Dose: 1 teaspoon (approx. 3 gr.) twice a day with warm water and honey between meals.

* Internal use is currently restricted by the FDA in the United States.

Case History 12

This woman came to me some years ago, before I stopped using manufactured Ayurvedic formulas. I have chosen her case because she was filled with many fibroids and had several cysts in her Fallopian tubes. This case demonstrates the power of self-healing. The patient's doctor recommended that she have a complete hysterectomy as soon as possible. She decided to try natural options, with her doctor's agreement, and got my name from a friend. She was a divorced, professional woman, 44 years old with three children. Her constitution was pitta and she had both a vata and pitta imbalance. Vata was strongly imbalanced and had moved into pitta. She had digestive problems, weak liver/gallbladder function, and an endocrine system that was quite disturbed. She was having a lot of pelvic pain, and it was almost impossible for her to have intercourse because of the pain. Her sleep was disturbed and she was dead tired.

She was under a lot of strain and stress in her personal life, which was compounded by the fact that she was caring for her aged mother at home. She was a dynamic and lively person who was looking at the psychological roots for her problems, both physically and emotionally. She was quite desperate when she came to me, so I put her on a strong treatment, which I do not recommend without supervision from a practitioner. First, I gave her a modern Ayurvedic liver formula called LIV-52, or Liver-52, made by the Himalayan Drug Company in Bangalore, India. There are many good liver formulas available, this is one that was available to me at the time. She took this formula for the year of treatment that she underwent with me.

Next, I treated her with the formula given in Table 29. She used this formula for two months and had some nausea from the detoxification of the liver and blood. We adjusted her formula for this, reducing the dose and raising it slowly. In two months, the pain she had been experiencing was completely gone. We then moved to tonics and strengthening her system because she was still tired most of the time. I gave her the simple formula shown in Table 30, while she continued with the Liv-52.

Table 29. Formula 1 for Case History 12

Dosha	(Ratio) Herb	Part of Plant	Effect on Metabolism	Effect on Dosha
Pitta	(3) Chaparral	plant	cooling	+V
	(2) Shatavari	root	cooling	+K
	(2) Haritaki	fruit	heating	=VPK
	(2) Triphala	fruits	warming	=VPK
	(1) Ginger	root	heating	+P

Table 30. Formula 2 for Case History 12

Dosha	(Ratio) Herb	Part of Plant	Effect on Metabolism	Effect on Dosha
Pitta	(2) Shatavari	root	cooling	+K
	(2) Licorice	root	cooling	+K
	(1) Triphala	fruits	warming	=VPK

The patient took 1 teaspoon of this formula daily for six months. During the course of this treatment, I gave her four pranic healing treatments of 45 minutes each to the pelvic area. In nine months, she felt her normal self again, but I advised her to continue with the liver formula until a year had passed. She had one more pranic treatment and saw me a year and a few weeks after our first meeting. Her doctor had said that "she was like a young girl." Needless to say, she was very happy and she is still healthy, more than three years later.

Tumors

In general, tumors should be treated as cysts. You can use the same formulas given in Tables 25, 26, 27 (see pages 161, 163, and 165). There is little difference, from the Ayurvedic point of view. Accumulation is always kapha in nature and can be caused by kapha itself, or by a constriction of vata.

What determines the treatment is the location (dhatu) and system (srota) involved. If the system is related to vata, treat vata primarily. If the system is a kapha system, treat kapha first. As stated before, pitta must always be considered because of the digestive relationship.

CHAPTER THIRTEEN

Other Problems

---

*That which shines as "Is" is Her Majesty the Absolute Consciousness.
Thus the universe is only the Self—the one and one only.*

—Tripura Rahasya

This chapter supplements other information given in this book. It covers other common problems and focuses on understanding the root of ailments—the reason for the disease to occur in the first place. Most of the treatments that follow aim at correcting the doshic imbalance that provides the environment for the "dis-ease" to take root. Some symptomatic remedies are given as well.

Cystitis

Cystitis, or urinary infections, happens to almost all women at some point. The weaker your kidneys are, the more prone to infection you will be. The controlling dosha of the kidneys is vata, with kapha second. Vata controls all elimination from the body. This function is under the direction of the apana vayu. The kidneys are also controlled by apana. Hence, the first place to begin treatment is to balance or strengthen the apana aspect of vata.

As always, determine your constitution and then identify the imbalance. The bladder and kidney pulse points are controlled by kapha, as kapha controls and is made from plasma, or body fluids. It is worth pointing out that "water" in the body is plasma, an oily liquid that is depleted by the consumption of excessive amounts of water. The kidneys become fatigued by the overconsumption of all liquids, including water. Those who tell you to drink a certain amount of water each day take a mechanical approach to the body and do not understand that a gallon of water a day can very quickly have detrimental effects for some constitutions. Vata women become tired and weak; kapha women bloat and hold excess fluid; pitta women seem to be able to process this amount without a problem.

Coffee, tea, soft drinks, and alcohol are all damaging to the kidney function and the water metabolism. Coffee and tea should be used in moderation; pops and soft drinks should not be used at all, because they rob your body of precious minerals and destroy the water metabolism. Alcohol should be taken only occasionally, because it dries out the kidneys and aggravates both vata and pitta. The excessive use of any of these drinks can cause chronic cystitis.

The point is that the health of your water metabolism, and by association the production of plasma and kapha, is dependent mostly on the state of the kidneys. As the kidneys are controlled by vata, and specifically by apana, any disturbance in the apana can eventually affect the kapha humor. This can happen with excess apana, which dries out kapha and the kidneys, by congested apana, which blocks kapha and increases bloating, or by apana aggravating the ranjaka pitta, which causes the urine to become full of toxins and can lead to infection. Cystitis is most often caused by apana aggravating ranjaka, which causes toxic infection. This can be carried up into the kidneys by apana if not treated.

A correct treatment approach drives both pitta (inflammation) and vata (disturbance) back to their proper roles and places in the body. Cold, bitter herbs are used to control pitta and demulcent, soothing herbs are used to treat vata. Diet and lifestyle should be addressed, since both improper eating and drinking habits can cause this problem. The frequently stated theory that excessive intercourse can cause cystitis is only half true. The doshas must be imbalanced for intercourse to have a negative effect on the urethra and bladder. Habitual consumption of the wrong liquids is more of a causal factor, because it sets up an environment that encourages infection by weakening the doshas and kidneys.

The formula given in Table 31 can be used to treat the symptoms of cystitis. Infuse 3 to 4 grams per cup of the formula in boiled water for 15 minutes and let cool to room temperature. Drink three times per day until urine is normal. If no infection is present, do not use the golden seal. If there is little urine, or difficulty urinating, add 3 parts of dandelion. If there is pain on urination, add 2 parts licorice. Do not use this formula for longer than two weeks. If the problem persists or is not fully solved, see a natural practitioner.

Table 31. Formula for Treating Cystitis

(Ratio) Herb	Part of Plant	Effect on Metabolism	Effect on Dosha
(3) Uva Ursi	plant	cooling	+V
(2) Gotu Kola	plant	cooling	=VPK
(2) Golden Seal	root	cooling	+V

Long-term treatment for chronic cystitis should balance your constitution. Treatment should last for one to two months. Table 32 gives some suggestions for balancing the water metabolisms of different constitutions.

Table 32. Formulas for Balancing Water Metabolism

Dosha	(Ratio) Herb	Part of Plant	Effect on Metabolism	Effect on Dosha
Vata	(3) Gotu Kola	plant	cooling	=VPK
	(2) Uva Ursi	plant	cooling	+V
	(2) Nettles	plant	cooling	+V
	(2) Valerian	root	heating	+P
	(2) Marshmallow	root	cooling	+K
	(2) Licorice	root	cooling	+K
	(1) Coriander	seed	cooling	=VPK
	(1) Fennel	seed	cooling	=VPK
	(1) Cumin	seed	cooling	=VPK
	(1) Ginger	root	heating	+P

Dose: 3 grams powder infused in 1 cup of boiled water 2 or 3 times a day.

Table 32. Formulas for Balancing Water Metabolism (cont.)

Pitta	(3) Gotu Kola	plant	cooling	=VPK
	(2) Uva Ursi	plant	cooling	+V
	(2) Dandelion	root	cooling	+V
	(2) Gentian	root	cooling	+V
	(2) Nettles	plant	cooling	+V
	(2) Marshmallow	root	cooling	+K
	(2) Licorice	root	cooling	+K
	(1) Fennel	seed	cooling	=VPK
	(1) Coriander	seed	cooling	=VPK
	(1) Cinnamon	bark	heating	+P

Dose: 3 grams powder infused in 1 cup of boiled water 2 or 3 times a day.

Kapha	(3) Gotu Kola	plant	cooling	=VPK
	(2) Uva Ursi	plant	cooling	+V
	(2) Dandelion	root	cooling	+V
	(2) Nettles	plant	cooling	+V
	(2) Valerian	root	heating	+P
	(1) Marshmallow	root	cooling	+K
	(1) Coriander	seed	cooling	=VPK
	(1) Fennel	seed	cooling	=VPK
	(1) Cumin	seed	cooling	=VPK
	(1) Ginger	root	heating	+P

Dose: 3 grams powder infused in 1 cup of boiled water 2 or 3 times a day.

Vulvodynia

Vulvodynia is the name now used for an unknown (at least from the Western standpoint) disorder that bothers many women. Vulvodynia means pain, itching, and/or burning sensations around the vulva. The most common form is called cyclic vulvodynia, because it comes and goes with the menstruation cycle. It has been linked to the LH cycle of menstruation.

According to Ayurveda, several things can create this situation. Those women who are vata, or have vata as part of their constitution, will be more prone to this disorder. Any constitutional type can suffer from this disorder, however, if there is a chronic imbalance of vata. Hence, natal constitution can make you more prone to it, but its actual cause is an imbalance of vata, in association with the bhrajaka pitta. This condition is best treated internally, through balancing the doshas, detoxifing the blood, balancing the endocrine function, and addressing emotional situations that have aggravated the nerves and vata in general.

Vata can easily be aggravated through mental stress or anxiety, which upsets the pituitary gland, via the hypothalamus, and disrupts endocrine harmony. Patients suffering from vulvodynia usually have some disturbance of vata in their lives, usually external, although it can result from the internalization of emotions as well. This source of vata disturbance should be found and corrected or the treatment may fail, since vata is the root cause of the problem.

If there is burning or itching associated with the condition, the bhrajaka pitta must be addressed as well. Bhrajaka can become disturbed by toxins in the blood or an aggravation of ranjaka pitta. Therefore, the blood should be detoxified and the digestive function balanced. Since agni must be low for this condition to exist, it should be increased to a proper level of function. The overall constitution should be balanced and a natural low-protein diet should be observed during treatment and for several months after.

Symptomatic, external treatment is limited in effect and does not correct the problem, although it can be used during the course of treatment to bring relief. Calendula cream is perhaps the best choice. Another skin remedy that may work for some women is the direct application of pure honey on the vulva.

The formulas given in Table 33 (see page 178) are for chronic conditions in each constitution and will generally work for all forms of vulvodynia. Suggested time of treatment is from three to six months, depending on how long the situation has existed and on the ability of the person to change external factors that may be causing the problem. The addition of 1 teaspoon of ghee will increase the effectiveness of these formulas for vata and pitta.

Table 33. Formulas for Treating Vulvodynia

Dosha	(Ratio) Herb	Part of Plant	Effect on Metabolism	Effect on Dosha
Vata	(3) Angelica	root	heating	+P
	(3) Agnus Castus	seed	heating	+P
	(3) Turmeric	root	heating	=VPK
	(2) Barberry	root	heating	+V
	(2) Licorice	root	cooling	+K
	(2) Nettles	plant	cooling	+V
	(2) Valerian	root	heating	+P
	(1) Calamus˙	root	heating	+P
	(1) Cumin	seed	cooling	=VPK
	(1) Fennel	seed	cooling	=VPK
	(1) Ginger	root	heating	+P

Dose: 1 teaspoon (approx. 3 gr.) twice a day with warm water and honey before meals. The addition of 1 teaspoon of ghee with the formula will increase its effectiveness.

Dosha	(Ratio) Herb	Part of Plant	Effect on Metabolism	Effect on Dosha
Pitta	(3) Agnus Castus	seed	heating	+P
	(3) Black Cohosh	root	cooling	+V
	(3) Barberry	root	heating	+V
	(2) Turmeric	root	heating	=VPK
	(2) Burdock	root	cooling	+V
	(2) Nettles	plant	cooling	+V
	(2) Licorice	root	cooling	+K
	(1) Cumin	seed	cooling	=VPK
	(1) Fennel	seed	cooling	=VPK
	(1) Cinnamon	bark	heating	+P

Dose: 1 teaspoon (approx. 3 gr.) twice a day with warm water and sugar before meals. The addition of 1 teaspoon of ghee with the formula will increase its effectiveness.

Table 33. Formulas for Treating Vulvodynia (cont.)

Kapha	(3) Angelica	root	heating	+P
	(3) Turmeric	root	heating	=VPK
	(2) Barberry	root	heating	+V
	(2) Agnus Castus	seed	heating	+P
	(2) Black Cohosh	root	cooling	+V
	(2) Myrrh	resin	heating	+P
	(2) Dandelion	root	cooling	+V
	(2) Nettles	plant	cooling	+V
	(1) Fenugreek	seed	heating	+P
	(1) Cumin	seed	cooling	=VPK
	(1) Ginger	root	heating	+P

Dose: 1 teaspoon (approx. 3 gr.) twice a day with warm water and honey before meals.

* Internal use is currently restricted by the FDA in the United States.

Pelvic Inflammatory Disease (PID) and Endometriosis

Inflammations of the uterus and pelvic area are pitta problems. Pitta is the focus of all treatment, yet vata must also be considered as both an emotional and movement source. Inflammations are moved and carried by vata, and the blood. They are often due to mental stress or disturbance caused by a disturbance of vata. However, treatment is primarily oriented to lower pitta to drive it from the blood and menstruation systems. There are often toxins present in this condition, because the toxins in the blood (pitta ama) feed the infection.

Kapha women are more prone to endometriosis than PID. Vata and pitta women are more prone to PID. In all of these conditions, however, and for all constitutions, pitta is the humor that has become imbalanced, since they are all inflammatory conditions. Generally, the blood and liver must be cleaned and their quality corrected, since they are the source of pitta in the body. Treatment must be supported by a vegetarian anti-pitta diet and a strict avoidance of all spices, alcohol, salt, and white sugars. Refined oils should be completely avoided as well. Since pitta is imbalanced, an emotional environment that is supportive to lower pitta is important. This means a quiet, noncompetitive, loving home that does not produce anger, frustration, irritations, or conflict.

In 1994, over five million women in the United States had or had had endometriosis. Seventy-five percent of these women were between 24 to 45. This is the pitta time of life. A hysterectomy is considered to be the best treatment by modern medicine. Ayurveda sees this as an imbalance in the immune system, stemming from low ojas, which also affects endocrine function. Therefore, the use of ojas-supporting herbs is important in balancing both the endocrine and immune systems.

I also believe this approach to be effective in treating salpingitis. The basic approach is the same and the formulas in Table 34 will, in many cases, work for both. The amount of golden seal should be increased by 1 unit in these formulas to treat salpingitis, depending on how acute the problem is when treatment begins. I suggest the formulas in Table 34 be taken for two to four months. This is a difficult problem and your health should be monitored by a professional if you are treating yourself. Each constitutional type should also take 4 grams of shatavari each day with warm cow's, soya, or rice milk to strengthen and rejuvenate the reproductive organs and ojas. This should be done for at least three to four months.

Table 34. Formulas for Treating PID and Endometriosis

Dosha	(Ratio) Herb	Part of Plant	Effect on Metabolism	Effect on Dosha
Vata	(3) Gotu Kola	plant	cooling	=VPK
	(3) Echinacea	root	cooling	+V
	(2) Myrrh	resin	heating	+P
	(2) Dandelion	root	cooling	+V
	(2) Turmeric	root	heating	=VPK

Table 34. Formulas for Treating PID and Endometriosis (cont.)

Vata (cont.)	(1) Golden Seal	root	cooling	+V
	(1) Barberry	root	heating	+V
	(1) Coriander	seed	cooling	=VPK
	(1) Fennel	seed	cooling	=VPK
	(¼) Saffron	flower	cooling	=VPK

Dose: 1 teaspoon (approx. 3 gr.) twice a day with warm water and honey before meals.

Pitta	(3) Gotu Kola	plant	cooling	=VPK
	(3) Echinacea	root	cooling	+V
	(2) Golden Seal	root	cooling	+V
	(2) Myrrh	resin	heating	+P
	(2) Dandelion	root	cooling	+V
	(2) Gentian	root	cooling	+V
	(2) Barberry	root	heating	+V
	(2) Turmeric	root	heating	=VPK
	(1) Fennel	seed	cooling	=VPK
	(1) Coriander	seed	cooling	=VPK
	(¼) Saffron	flower	cooling	=VPK

Dose: 1 teaspoon (approx. 3 gr.) twice a day with warm water and sugar before meals. The addition of 1 teaspoon of ghee with the formula will increase its effectiveness.

Kapha	(3) Gotu Kola	plant	cooling	=VPK
	(3) Echinacea	root	cooling	+V
	(2) Golden Seal	root	cooling	+V
	(2) Turmeric	root	heating	=VPK
	(2) Barberry	root	heating	+V
	(2) Myrrh	resin	heating	+P
	(2) Dandelion	root	cooling	+V
	(2) Uva Ursi	plant	cooling	+V
	(1) Fennel	seed	cooling	=VPK
	(1) Coriander	seed	cooling	=VPK
	(¼) Saffron	flower	cooling	=VPK

Dose: 1 teaspoon (approx. 3 gr.) twice a day with warm water and honey before meals.

Case History 13

A woman came to me with a chronic case of endometriosis. She was 39 years old and had had chronic menstrual problems her whole life. In her early 20s, she was diagnosed as having endometriosis. She had very strong pain before, during, and after menstruation. She reluctantly took pain medication. Recently, the periods of pain had increased to encompass three weeks out of each month, which was why she had come to me for help. Intercourse was very difficult and even painful on occasion. Her constitution was kapha/vata, with an imbalance of pitta and vata. The vata had moved into pitta and caused the beginning of the problem when she was a young woman. This was not corrected and endometriosis resulted. Diagnosis showed a chronic imbalance of vata and pitta with a toxic blood condition. I suggested that she take the formula in Table 35 for a month.

Table 35. Formula 1 for Case History 13

Dosha	(Ratio) Herb	Part of Plant	Effect on Metabolism	Effect on Dosha
Kapha/ Vata	(3) Turmeric	root	heating	=VPK
	(3) Dandelion	root	cooling	+V
	(2) Barberry	root	heating	+V
	(2) Gentian	root	cooling	+V
	(2) Asparagus	root	cooling	+K
	(2) Echinacea	root	cooling	+V
	(2) Raspberry	plant	cooling	+V
	(1) Myrrh	resin	heating	+P
	(1) Golden Seal	root	cooling	+V
Dose: 2 "00" capsules twice a day.				

The patient took 2 "00" capsules of this formula three times per day before eating. After one month, she felt much better, had less pain, and felt more energetic. Her tongue had cleared of toxins and the blood was about 60 percent less toxic. She was still experiencing pain, but for shorter periods of time and less strongly. During this time, she also began with a treatment of shatavari at 4 grams per day. At this point, I recommended that she change to the formula given in Table 36 for four months. She took 2 "00" capsules twice a day between meals for four months. When I saw her four months later, she was experiencing pain only two days before her menstruation and that pain was bearable without medication. She felt well and was very happy. She still continues to take shatavari, on my advice, and continues to improve.

Table 36. Formula 2 for Case History 13

DOSHA	(RATIO) HERB	PART OF PLANT	EFFECT ON METABOLISM	EFFECT ON DOSHA
Kapha/ Vata	(3) Cramp Bark	bark	heating	+P
	(3) Raspberry	plant	cooling	+V
	(2) Agnus Castus	seed	heating	+P
	(2) Dandelion	root	cooling	+V
	(2) Barberry	root	heating	+V
	(2) Turmeric	root	heating	=VPK
	(2) Gentian	root	cooling	+V
	(1) Myrrh	resin	heating	+P
	(1) Cinnamon	bark	heating	+P

Cancers

I do not have a lot of experience in treating cancer, so I can only give the general Ayurvedic viewpoint on the subject. Perhaps this will be helpful for women who are confronted with this grave problem.

Ayurveda considers cancer to involve all three humors and toxins. Ojas (the result of all tissue production) is low, affecting immunity. Generally, it is thought that toxins must be present for a substantial period of time in order for ojas to become low and the doshas to become imbalanced.

There is often a dietary deficiency. Many studies have linked cancer to diets high in proteins, fat, and processed foods. Some evidence exists that shows that milk products—especially low-fat dairy products—can cause cancer in certain people. Many chemicals in our food chain and daily lives are known to cause cancer.

However, the main point of Ayurveda is that the metabolism and the three humors have been out of balance for some time before a cancerous growth can begin in the body. Moreover, the mind must be disturbed. This disturbance can reflect how you relate to yourself. Some researchers are of the opinion that a negative self-image can be a definite contributing factor in developing cancer.

The best steps you can take are to become a strict vegetarian, eating no animal products, and buying only organic foods. You must balance all three doshas and increase agni. Deficient agni is a major cause of all wasting diseases. When the digestion is functioning well and is able to digest correctly, immunomodulating herbs can be taken to strengthen the immune system. These herbs should increase ojas, your fundamental energy source. Daily exercise and meditation are very important factors. All of these steps should be taken before submitting yourself to chemotherapy or surgery.

On a deeper level, Ayurveda considers cancers to be foreign beings in the body. For these "beings" to take root, there must be a break in the life-force, or refined state of vata, known as prana. This prana is the link between the body, personality, mental function, and the soul. It is the soul that is going to heaven or reincarnating (depending on your personal beliefs). It is the prana that is holding the body to the soul. From the Ayurvedic point of view, cancer cannot take hold in the body if this link is strong. There must be some conscious or unconscious break in the very desire to live. The will to live is the "tangible link" that we have with prana. Somehow, this link has become disturbed and the "other being"—cancer—has taken root in the body. This is a poor attempt to explain some of the more subtle functions of the prana and how it relates to the individualized consciousness manifest in the temple of the body. Also, if the temple is abused or rejected, the link with prana is weakened.

A happy life is the best prevention for cancer, or for that matter, any disease. Dr. Deepak Chopra is very experienced in cancer treatment and can benefit women with cancer. The address for The Chopra Center for Well-Being is listed in Appendix 5. Also see Susun Weed's book on breast cancer in the bibliography.

Hysterectomy

If you have had a hysterectomy, the best thing you can do is use tonic herbs to strengthen your body and support your other hormone-producing organs. If you haven't had a hysterectomy, the best thing you can do is not to have one—unless your life is threatened by cancer.

In a study done from 1987 to 1989, an insurance company found that at least one-third of the hysterectomies performed during that time were not needed. By age 60, one-third of all women in the United States have had a hysterectomy! In 1995, over 750,000 were performed. One-third of those were for fibroids, a condition that's possible to treat using herbs, diet, and lifestyle. Some years before, 13,000 hysterectomies were performed to cure PMS. While these figures are common knowledge, what is not generally known is that up to half of all hysterectomies performed are accompanied by complications. This means you have a 50 percent chance that something else can go wrong. This is *not* a simple operation, nor is it without risk, by any means. Most of the medical profession is of the opinion that the only justification for a hysterectomy is a life-threatening situation, like cancer of the uterus.

This book has given alternative solutions to all of the problems that are used to justify the need for a hysterectomy. It is thought by many natural practitioners that only about 5 percent of all hysterectomies need be performed at all. Public attention has shifted in this direction over the last few years, and progress is being made in educating women to options and alternatives. Following the guidelines given in this book should help prevent the need for a hysterectomy.

As mentioned above, if you have had a hysterectomy, Ayurveda advises that you use the menopause formula to support your endocrine system. This is a better option than taking estrogen therapy, since both ERT and HRT have been implicated in causing cancer. Follow the formulas given in chapter 11 to support and nourish your body naturally. This will increase your quality of life and help you remain active and vital.

CHAPTER FOURTEEN

Nutrition as a Healing Power

I am the abstract intelligence where from the cosmos originates,
whereon it flourishes, and wherein it resolves, like the images in a mirror.
The ignorant know me as the gross universe, whereas the wise
feel me as their own pure being eternally glowing as "I-I" within.

—Tripura Rahasya

The medical evidence is overwhelming: A long term diet based on animal foods is detrimental to the human body. Any person who has explored this subject without bias and with personal experience has converted to a plant-based diet. One of the latest world authorities to follow this trend is Dr. Benjamin Spock.

Shortly before his death in 1998, Dr. Spock revised his world-famous book, *Baby and Child Care*, to recommend a diet based solely on plants after age 2. Of course, that means adults as well. While Spock's conclusions have come under fire from certain quarters, they are in keeping with several decades of medical research. Dr. Spock is quoted as saying that he wanted to be at the forefront of the new nutritional programs that would emerge in the next twenty years. This is a bold statement from one of America's medical icons.

A well-known author, John Robbins, quotes the findings of medical research in his books. These studies point to the age between weaning and 4 years old as the time when it is potentially most damaging for humans to consume high-protein animal foods. The effects of a high-protein diet in the formative years can create food sensitivities, allergies, immune suppression, obesity, and other diseases. This is an even more radical view than that of Dr. Spock, yet one that has a scientific basis.

Moreover, Dr. Spock is not the only world authority to take such a stance in recent years. Another famous man, Dr. T. Colin Campbell, Professor of Nutritional Sciences at Cornell University and a former senior science advisor to the American Institute of Cancer Research, has also made the switch to a plant-based diet. Dr. Campbell was the director of the most comprehensive study ever done on the relationship between diet and disease. The twenty-year study, called the China-Oxford-Cornell Study, compared the diet and disease tendencies of cultures and groups of people. Among other things, the study concluded that excessive animal protein is the root cause of many chronic, terminal diseases common in modern society. Dr. Campbell became a vegetarian during the course of the study because its evidence was overwhelmingly clear. Different groups have called the study one-sided because Dr. Campbell is now a vegetarian. Campbell states, however, that the evidence came first. Having a truly scientific mind, he simply accepted the evidence and switched his own diet and that of his family.[1]

It has been mentioned several times in this book that a high-protein diet (i.e., one based on animal foods) is detrimental to health and actually causes many diseases or problems. Without going into detail, the primary reason for this is the protein itself. Protein molecules are extremely large. They provide a structural element to cells and generally provide the structure upon which the whole body is built. The body does not store protein and so needs to have a continuous supply. The body actually needs very little protein, however, and easily gets enough protein if the overall calorie intake is sufficient. This means that, if you are taking

---

[1] See these books for more information on Dr. Campbell's work: John Robbins, *Diet for a New World* (New York: Avon Books, 1992) p. 66; J. Chen, et al., *Diet, Lifestyle, and Mortality in China: A Study of the Characteristics of 65 Countries* (Oxford University Press, Cornell University Press, and the China People's Medical Publishing House, 1990).

enough calories, you are getting enough protein, provided you are not living on sugar, jellies, and denatured foods.

The protein molecule is made up of smaller units which we call amino acids. When we consume amino acids in foods, they then go to build the actual protein molecules. It is alternately tragic and hilarious that the principle reason "professionals" give for using an animal-based diet is its high protein content. It is precisely this very high protein content, however, that causes disease. Dr. Ballentine explains the problem like this in his classic book on nutrition:

> Any amino acids which are not needed for the construction of new protein molecules can be burned as fuel. This is not a "clean burning" fuel, however, since the nitrogen atom itself cannot be oxidized by the body. Proteins are like bricks. Although one might use them to make a fireplace, he certainly wouldn't attempt to use them as fuel for the fire; they require too much heat and leave too much residue. The nitrogen fragment of the amino acid molecule and the remains of other protein substances make up urea and uric acid. When the kidneys are unable to excrete all of the uric acid through the urine, it may accumulate in the tissues and joints and crystallize, producing protein toxicity.[2]

Whether or not you want to acknowledge the evidence is another matter. It has been clear for over a decade that vegetarians live longer, have fewer diseases, and enjoy a better quality of life in their later years. There are two factors that need to be clarified with regard to nutrition and diet in general. These two factors must be understood in approaching any kind of diet—plant or animal. The first factor is the

---

[2] Dr. Rudolph Ballentine, *Diet and Nutrition: A Holistic Approach* (Honesdale, PA: Himalayan International Institute, 1978), pp. 113–114.

presumption that the biochemical model of nutrition is valid and that it works. The second includes the methods of agriculture, transportation, and the presentation and preparation of food that are currently used in today's society.

The main fault in modern nutrition is that it uses a biochemical model, which we demonstrated earlier is quite limited in approach and understanding. Granted, the understanding of the chemical structures is clear, at least within the known factors. However, the interaction of nutrients in the body and with each other is not clearly understood, even though certain people would like you to think otherwise. The "synergy" of food and its interaction in the whole body is still largely a mystery. The biochemical model presumes that dividing up food into many chemicals, playing around with them, and giving them to a living human will have the same effect as eating whole foods occurring in a natural state. This logic is flawed. Following it can incur secondary effects, or even primary effects, when used without intelligence, as some people in America do today. One simply has to observe the huge number of obese children and adults in our society to prove this point.

While this whole question will be debated for many years, the eventual outcome will undoubtedly be that the biochemical model does not work for nutrition or medicine. It will take some time for this to become mainstream practice, because there are difficult factors to overcome, like economic realities and the education of the medical community in nutrition. Understand clearly that your doctor is not trained in nutrition and may know less about it than you do. This fact alone—that nutrition is not taught beyond a chemical understanding in medical schools—is enough to indicate the total absurdity of the biochemical approach. It is hard to believe that an intelligent person cannot see that what is consumed each day over many years will be the principal factor in deciding health or disease.

The second factor, the actual quality of our food, is equally important. The fact is that, unless you are eating organic foods, all your foods are now full of hormones and tissue-altering chemicals. There is no level of the food chain that is immune to this influence. Even "organic" foods have traces of hormones and poison chemicals in them, because the whole water system is affected. These facts are not disputed by the scientific community. The only question is how much of these foreign substances the body can eliminate and at what level the body becomes unable to eliminate them. These levels are determined on averages. After studies have been performed, a certain level is considered to be "safe." Once more, I do not consider myself an average, so I do not accept this kind of logic. The levels will invariably be too high or too low for many people. You may be one of the ones who is overly sensitive. I feel that any level of toxins is too high—yet I live in a large city and so must adjust to the reality of modern society. This does not mean that we have to accept the flawed logic and justifications of the current medical and nutritional communities.

Modern agricultural methods have altered the food chain and thus the nutrients available to the human body. This is primarily due to the use of chemical fertilizers and pesticides. Most vegetables in a natural environment provide traces of vitamin B_{12} around their roots and stems due to the fungi living in dirt. The earth itself is alive with fungi and bacteria that are responsible for the transformation of many fundamental components in nutrition. The natural bacteria around these roots provide the one nutrient that biochemical nutritionists claim does not exist in the plant kingdom. They are right. If you are buying and eating food from your local supermarket, that food is missing half the natural nutrients it would have if you grew it in your backyard without pesticides. However, they are wrong if the whole plant is considered and it is grown organically (or simply in a nonchemical environment).

Another factor is that food is harvested far too early and transported to markets, leaving it with little taste and often less nutrient content. Moreover, storage and packaging also reduce nutrient content, because agricultural products are often sprayed with substances that make them look better and last longer.

Doctor Ballentine's book, *Diet and Nutrition*, is a classic in the holistic nutritional field and is written with knowledge and integrity.[3] It is worth reading if you wish to have a better understanding of the biochemical model of nutrition as seen by a scientist (i.e., one who is open-minded and observes). His book also gives an introduction to Ayurvedic nutrition and provides a meeting point between the two systems for professionals or interested people. Diet is important. This is an aspect of your health over which you can take control and change, thereby changing your overall health and longevity and creating a positive healing power around which to center your treatments.

Ayurvedic Nutrition

Ayurveda has a very different vision of diet and nutrition. The primary concern of Ayurveda is your ability to digest food. The second is to eat foods that balance your constitution and do not cause metabolic imbalance. The third is to eat foods that are as close as possible to their natural state. Finally, Ayurveda says that you must eat and then give ample time for the body to digest what you have taken in before you add more food. Failure to do this can overwork the digestive system, create toxins, and shorten your life span.

Absurd trends develop every so often in fashion and in nutrition. The latest trend, which advocates eating constantly throughout the day, is a sure way to shorten your life by twenty years. If you think that your body enjoys being on a constant marathon, continue to eat all day. Just because animals can do it does not make it appropriate for humans. Look at the life-span of a deer or gazelle. The fad of

---

[3] Dr. Rudolph Ballentine, *Diet and Nutrition: A Holistic Approach* (Honesdale, PA: Himalayan International Institute, 1978).

"grazing" is just that—a fad. It will overwork your digestion and not allow it to rest. This will tax the digestive organs and they will become imbalanced, resulting in toxins and the beginning of the disease process. If you are hungry all the time, or feel the need to munch between meals, this indicates an imbalance in the metabolism. The point is to find the root of the problem—malabsorption, hormonal imbalance, an overload of toxins, or simply low agni.

So what is *agni*? Agni is the actual process of transformation in the digestion. It is often called the actual ability to digest and/or assimilate something. So if your agni is low, your ability to absorb and digest is low. Agni also exists in the tissues and the mind. It is the principle that digests or transforms everything in the body. The digestive agni is the chief, or principal, agni in the body. The other forms of agni are related to it and can be determined to some extent by the state of the main digestive agni. *Low agni is behind all accumulation of toxins in the body and most digestive disorders.*

Therefore, the first consideration of nutrition in Ayurveda begins, not with what you are eating, but with what you have the ability to digest. The logic behind this is, of course, quite solid. You may be eating the best organic food available and still feel tired and have low energy. This is because your agni—your ability to digest it—is not sufficient for the foods that you are consuming, whether animal or vegetable. Low agni is behind many dietary and metabolic problems. It can eventually lead to a breakdown of the digestive process and create diseases like obesity, arthritis, or certain forms of diabetes. It is behind all forms of chronic disease. It is also behind all nutrient deficiencies and is linked to many food allergies. So before anything else, look at the level of agni in your body, then begin to make dietary changes.

The second consideration—balancing the constitution through food—is accomplished by a profound system. Ayurveda uses a method of understanding the five elements in both the body and food. In the body, we use the three doshas—vata, pitta, and kapha—because each of them controls two of the five elements. With food, however, we need a more precise system. Ayurveda, therefore, uses six classifications to understand all the possible element combinations in food. The elements in food will tend to balance or imbalance the doshas by reducing or increasing them respectively. This system is called the Six Tastes.

The concept behind the use of the Six Tastes is that each taste provides a necessary item for the proper functioning of the metabolism. Therefore, meals should be constructed to include all of the Six Tastes found in food:

Sweet or bland;   Pungent or hot;
Salty or salty;   Bitter or tart;
Sour or acidic;   Astringent.

When a diet includes all of these tastes, it becomes "balanced"—not in the biochemical sense, but in the overall "synergy" of the metabolism. This concept is very profound and it would be a mistake to discard it as simplistic. To learn it is not necessarily easy, to really understand it is difficult. We are saved, however, by many great Ayurvedic doctors who have figured out the nature of different foods for us. The most notable of these doctors in modern times are Drs. Vasant Lad and David Frawley. Their students have continued to adapt much of the traditional information to our modern diet. This allows us to use the system itself without having to understand more than its fundamentals, which I have given above. Table 37 shows the relationships between the different tastes and the doshas.

Table 37. Effect of the Six Tastes on the Doshas

Humor	Increases	Decreases
Vata	bitter/pungent/astringent	sweet/sour/salty
Pitta	sour/salty/pungent	sweet/bitter/astringent
Kapha	sweet/sour/salty	pungent/bitter/astringent

The six tastes exist in all foods and substances. Moreover, every food has all of the tastes. Sometimes the tastes are latent, meaning you cannot actually taste them. Normally, one taste will dominate the others, which generates the classifications that you find in books. The tastes also exist in pure or complex forms. The pure forms will imbalance you faster than the complex forms. Generally, you should use the complex forms in our daily diet and only use the pure forms in small amounts and occasionally. For example, the use of alcohol will imbalance the doshas quickly—like a "hangover"—while the use of yogurt in excess will take several days or weeks to imbalance the doshas. Table 38 gives examples of the different forms.

Table 38. The Six Tastes in Pure and Complex Forms

Taste	Pure Form	Form
Sweet	sugars	complex carbohydrates, grains
Sour	alcohol	yogurt, lemon
Salty	table salt	soy sauce, seaweed
Pungent	cayenne pepper	mild spice, cinnamon, onions
Bitter	gentian, aloe	rhubarb, leafy dark-green plants
Astringent	unripe bananas	pomegranate, cranberries

The third factor in good nutrition is eating what grows around you. This is the food that is easiest for your body to digest. It also means that your local food will follow the seasons. Imported food will usually have little to do with the state of the doshas moving in nature (i.e., the seasons) and will therefore tend to imbalance the doshas in the body. Eating what is grown naturally, in season, and current with your cultural upbringing is important, according to Ayurveda.

The fourth factor is eating twice or three times per day and allowing food to be completely digested before eating more. This has been discussed briefly above. It is logical to conclude that, by never giving your digestive system a rest, you can cause it to break down sooner than if you gave it a rest each day. At the very least, do not overload it with continuous input. You should feel hungry before you eat. If you are hungry all the time then your metabolism is not working properly. In this case, you should consult a qualified Ayurvedic practitioner.

Diet by Humor

Table 39 gives the basic foods that balance each dosha (see page 198). This table is not comprehensive, but it is a good place to start. Following these suggestions the majority of the time can create a positive force in your body to balance your constitution. Seventy to 80 percent compliance will bring health. Occasionally eating foods not on the list will not affect your health, provided you do not consume them more than 20 percent of the time. For example, in each week you eat 21 meals (3 meals a day X 7 days). Seventeen of these meals represent 80 percent of your diet; and four of them represent 20 percent of your diet. This should *not* be taken to mean that in four dinners out of seven you can indulge in chocolate-covered eggplant. It means that, if, a few times a week, you eat other food items that are not on your list, the effect will be negligible. The bibliography provides more information on Ayurvedic nutrition. See especially the books of Amedea Morningstar. Remember: the primary question is whether or not you can you digest the foods on your list.

In general, you should use the diet that lowers your constitutional humor. However, in cases of imbalance or aggravation, anyone can use any of the above diets to control an imbalance. If any doubt persists, consult an Ayurvedic practitioner. In general, vata types or people with high vata do not digest raw foods well. If you have an imbalance of vata, avoid raw foods. This doesn't mean you have to cook things to death; lightly steamed is already better than raw.

Mixed constitutions should follow the diet that relates to the season. For example, a pitta/kapha person should eat a diet that balances pitta from the middle of spring to the beginning of fall, and then eat a diet that balances kapha the rest of the time. Remember, vata controls fall and early winter, kapha controls late winter and early spring, and pitta controls late spring and summer. Balance your diet according to the seasons if you are a mixed type.

The concept of nutrition in Ayurveda uses the Six Tastes to balance foods. With understanding, we can use different foods, spices, and combinations of foods and spices to change the qualities of food. That means that, if a food you like is not on your list, don't despair! Instead, learn how to modify its qualities so that you can eat it without imbalancing your system. This is the beauty of Ayurveda. Ayurveda is not a rigid system. If it is being presented in a "yes" and "no" fashion, the person doing so has not understood the true method of using the Six Tastes and their underlying elements. I strongly encourage those of you who are interested in food, or those of you suffering from a chronic illness, to learn more.

Another major misconception about Ayurvedic nutrition is that you have to eat Indian food. Ayurvedic nutrition has nothing to do with eating any specific kind of food. It is a system of understanding the "energies" of food. For example, I do about half the cooking at home and I make an Indian dish about once every few months or even less—yet I cook with Ayurvedic principles all the time.

Table 39. Diets for Lowering the Three Doshas

DOSHA	FRUITS	VEGETABLE	GRAINS	ANIMALS	BEANS	NUTS	DAIRY	OILS
Vata	sweet fruits apricots avocados bananas berries citrus (not sour) melons peaches	cooked veggies asparagus carrots cucumber green beans leeks olives onions sweet potatoes pumpkins squash	oats all kinds of rice wheat	chicken turkey duck fish seafood eggs	go easy on the beans adzuki mung (or moong) soy milk tofu (cooked)	all nuts are OK	all dairy is OK	all oils are OK
Pitta	sweet fruits apples avocados berries dates figs grapes melons pears plums	sweet & bitter veggies artichoke asparagus broccoli brussels sprouts cabbage corn cauliflower leafy greens	barley cooked oats basmati rice white rice wheat	chicken turkey rabbit eggs	adzuki beans black beans chickpeas kidney beans lima mung pinto soybeans & products tofu	coconut	butter cottage cheese soft cheeses ghee milk	Coconut oil olive oil sunflower oil soy oil

Table 39. Diets for Lowering the Three Doshas (cont.)

Dosha	Fruits	Vegetable	Grains	Animals	Beans	Nuts	Dairy	Oils
Pitta (cont.)		lettuce mushrooms potatoes squash						
Kapha	bitter & astringent fruits apricots berries cherries cranberries peaches pears persimmons pomegranate prunes raisins	pungent & bitter veggies asparagus beets broccoli cabbage carrots cauliflower corn eggplant garlic leafy greens leeks mushrooms onions peas peppers spinach sprouts turnips	barley buckwheat corn quinoa rye	chicken turkey boiled eggs	adzuki beans lima beans mung beans navy beans pinto beans split peas white beans	no nuts	no dairy	almond oil corn oil sunflower oil

Using Food Medicinally

Using diet to balance the humors—eating foods that prevent humors from accumulating—is medical in approach. Ayurveda considers the best medicine to be food. The right use of food should be used to support all the formulas given in the previous chapters. Without the foundation of a diet that balances your constitution, you may not achieve good results, or your results may be slower. *This point cannot be emphasized enough.*

We can understand this by looking once more at the five vayus of the vata humor. As discussed over and over in this book, vata is the main cause of disease and is behind all gynecological problems to some extent. The main source of raw material that becomes vata in the body is food. Living, natural food contains large amounts of prana. This prana is absorbed in the digestive process—primarily in the colon by the apana vayu—and is converted to vata. When vata is in balance the food prana is purified by vata and becomes a refined state of prana in the body. This refined state of prana provides the basis of all three humors and their refined states of ojas (from kapha), tejas (from pitta), and prana (from vata). When these three are in balance, we have good health, physically and mentally.

When vata is disturbed, the absorption of the prana in food is disrupted. This in turn affects the production of all the doshas. That affects the refined states of ojas, tejas, and prana, which lowers our vitality, immunity, and mental flexibility—and thus our overall health. Hence, the correct absorption of prana from the food is the basis of good health and proper nutrition. Agni, in the small intestine, prepares food and prana to be assimilated in the colon. This is why agni is so important. If agni is not functioning well, toxins accumulate in the colon and impair the absorption of prana, affecting all of the doshas and our health.

Therefore, if you are eating junk food, processed food, or devitalized food, you are taking in very little prana, and what you do take in will be of an inferior quality. Microwave ovens also reduce the pranic content in food and should be avoided. This once more places the emphasis on eating foods as close as possible to their natural state. Water is another major source of prana and the kidneys are vata organs. Here again, intake of detrimental liquids, like soft drinks, will derange the kidneys, and so vata, and eventually affect the amount of prana taken in by the body. Manufactured drinks and liquids do not have prana in them. Water and fruit juice do.

One point that is worth mentioning concerns dairy products. While much of the information presented here about animal products is somewhat negative, Ayurveda has a good view of dairy products. Natural dairy, that is. Ayurveda asserts that a cow represents the mother, or Mother Nature. She always provides more than what is needed. A cow has four udders, one for the baby calf, one for the farmer, one for the guest that may come, and one for the worship of the divine. From this point of view, the cow was not only a source of nutrition, but integral to the relationship of Earth and the divine. Each family had their own cow and looked on it, not only as a source of wealth, but as a gift from and an incarnation of the Divine Mother.

In today's Western world (and in much of modern India), the cow does not symbolize these things, especially not the relationship with the Divine Mother. Therefore, it is important to understand the Ayurvedic view of milk products from this standpoint. Modern dairy farming treats cows in a manner that changes the quality of the milk. The additional use of hormones and antibiotics renders the milk poisonous. As if that were not enough, pasteurizing the milk changes the enzyme structure in a way that makes it almost impossible to digest. Low-fat milk products have been linked to a number of different diseases (including some cancers) and are to be avoided at all cost. Whole milk is much better for the body because the cholesterol in it can be digested, whereas the cholesterol in "low-fat" products cannot. This makes it obvious that the milk products that are spoken of in Ayurveda are not what you are getting from your local supermarket.

Ayurveda has certain understandings about dairy as well. Milk should always be organic (the cow should be fed organic food and not given any chemicals), bought raw, and boiled immediately. Let it cool and then refrigerate it. This changes the enzyme structure in such a way as to make it more digestible. Milk should be taken warm, never cold and never frozen, as that increases its mucous-forming properties and encourages the formation of toxins. It should not be fermented, as is cheese. Fermentation also encourages the formation of toxins. Finally, spices like cinnamon and cardamom should be added to the milk to make it even more digestible.

If used in this way, milk products are very beneficial for the body. Ayurveda considers milk to nourish all seven tissues (dhatus) and to be especially good for the reproductive organs. Most rejuvenating herbs are given with milk or ghee. However, this same product, grown and produced in today's manner, is potentially damaging to the body. Animals are not machines. If they are given respect and love, they can give food that is nourishing to humans. If not, their products, laced with hormones and antibiotics, can be a source of disease. Hence, it is not milk that is questionable, but how we receive it from the cow.

Liver-Detox Formulas

Several times in this book, I have mentioned that the liver should be detoxified. In Table 40, I have included a simple detox formula for each of the three humors, even though the liver is primarily a pitta organ (see page 203). All of the constitutions can benefit from liver detoxification, because our diets tend to contain many pitta-aggravating foods, such as fried foods, poor-quality oils, red meats, alcohol, and sugar. Care should be given whenever any form of detoxification is being done not to go too quickly. Going too rapidly is contraindicated in all forms of detoxification in Ayurveda. The body does not like shocks. It is far more effective to slowly detoxify the liver (or body).

Signs that the liver is being detoxified too fast include headaches, skin rashes, sluggishness, nausea, fever, and hot emotions like anger. Follow the recommended doses. These formulas will also increase agni, which is an important part of Ayurvedic detoxification. Agni, if strong, will burn up toxins that are released, preventing any side effects like those given above. These formulas are best taken in the spring, to cleanse excessive pitta from the liver and clear toxins that have accumulated there. For all constitutional types, oils should be avoided, as should fried foods and sugar while using these formulas. The use of ghee can help promote liver function and is known to help the action of bitter, liver-cleansing herbs.

Table 40. Formulas for Detoxifying the Liver

Dosha	(Ratio) Herb
Vata	(2) Turmeric (2) Barberry (2) Dandelion (1) Asafoetida (1) Cumin (1) Fennel (1) Dry Ginger
Dose: ½ teaspoon in warm water before eating twice a day for 7 days. Then increase to 1 level teaspoon for 7 days; then increase to 1 "normal" teaspoon for 14 days. Use as little water as possible as the formula does not taste good!	

Table 40. Formulas for Detoxifying the Liver (cont.)

Pitta	(3) Gentian (3) Barberry (2) Turmeric (2) Dandelion (2) Gotu Kola (1) Cumin (1) Fennel (1) Coriander

Dose: ½ teaspoon in warm water before eating twice a day for 7 days. Then increase to 1 level teaspoon for 7 days; then increase to 1 "normal" teaspoon for 14 days. Use as little water as possible as the formula does not taste good!

Or use aloe gel alone: 1 tablespoon morning and night for 7 days; then increase to 2 tablespoons twice a day; then take ¼ cup in the morning for 14 days.

Kapha	(3) Turmeric (2) Barberry (2) Dandelion (1) Gentian (1) Cumin (1) Fennel (1) Black Pepper (1) Dry Ginger

Dose: ½ teaspoon in warm water before eating twice a day for 7 days. Then increase to 1 level teaspoon for 7 days; then increase to 1 "normal" teaspoon for 14 days. Use as little water as possible as the formula does not taste good!

May all beings be at peace and may the Divine Mother once more be respected by every human being as the source of everything. Namaskar! Sri Tripura!

> *Such illumination is Her Transcendental Majesty Tripura, the Supreme. She is called Brahma in the Vedas, Vishnu by the Vaishnavites, Siva by the Saivites, and Sakti by the Saktas. There is indeed nothing but She.*

—Tripura Rahasya

Appendix 1

Getting Off Pharmaceutical Medications

This information is not meant to replace professional medical advice. It is presented as a supplement to the information presented in this book. This information represents my own professional experience and may not be acceptable or legal in your state or country. If you are in doubt, consult your medical professional.

In chapter 6, a lengthy discussion was given on the effects of synthetic products on the body. This is a supplement to that information showing how I have helped women to stop using synthetic pharmaceutical products without experiencing adverse symptoms. Your individual situation may be different. If in doubt consult a professional.

The body does not like shocks. Stopping a medication suddenly may have adverse effects on your system, in spite of whatever adverse effects the medication itself might be having on you. The best way around this is to begin taking herbs and, after one month of taking the herbs, cut your dosage of medication in half. After the second month, again cut your medication in half. Continue this until it is impractical to "half it" any more. This usually takes three to four months—enough time for the body to adapt.

The general rule is that dietary or herbal changes need three months to effect a real change in your metabolism. Of course, high doses or treatment of acute problems (symptoms) do not fall under this category. This applies to different eating habits to change overall health (balance your constitution) or herbal formulas to correct imbalances in your constitution. Most of the formulas in this book are designed to work on a long-term basis, correcting the metabolic balance we call the constitution.

This means that, if you take an herbal formula for a period of three months, you will be changing the habitual function of the body. As the body has become habituated to synthetic products, it needs a period of "reeducation." This should be done gradually. Normally, I suggest that women not change their medication for the first month, but rather give time for the herbs to work. Depending on the medication, the dose can then be lowered. This is almost always safe for any kind of hormonal supplement or antidepressant, provided the antidepressant has not been used for more than a year, or two at the most. In this situation the liver, kidneys, and adrenals suffer and must be strengthened before attempting to remove the medication.

Other medications should be addressed individually and with your doctor. I am mainly concerned here with the products used especially by women, i.e., hormones and antidepressants. I cannot give advice on other kinds of medication, as they are beyond my field of knowledge. It is best to work with an herbalist and a doctor together. Also, if you have a heart condition or life-threatening disease, this advice is not for you.

An example of this is to use the formula for vata depression to withdraw from an antidepressant. Begin with the herbs for a month. After a month, cut the four pills you were taking to two per day. For the second month, take the herbs and two pills. At the beginning of the third month, take only one pill during the early evening. At the beginning of the fourth month, stop taking any medication other than the herbal formula. You must continue to take the herbs for another three months after you stop taking the medication. This means six months total for the herbal formula—three with medication and three without. If at any time you feel you need to take more medication, do so. When you are able, reduce the dose again.

Some herbalists are afraid to give this advice for fear of lawsuits or problems with the medical community. Some medications may, sometimes, react to some herbs. It is always good to ask your doctor whether a particular medication has any known reaction to herbs. It is best to avoid problems beforehand.

Vata people will have the most difficulty actually getting off medications. They need support and should be given guidance, because their bodies tend to be addicted to the chemicals. Pitta people can withdraw from medication the most easily, because they have determination. They may, however, be impatient and want to do it too fast. Kapha people will need a support system (a group of people is best for them) to stop their attachment to the feeling of the medication and emotional dependence on it.

The longer you have taken a product, the more slowly you should go in stopping it. The more dependent you are on it, the more care you should take.

Stopping the birth control pill can bring great relief, or great disruption, to your now-dependent endocrine system. Vata women will have the greatest problem in adjusting without the pill. Using the premenopause formula (see chapter 10) for your constitutional type will help to balance your hormone system and elevate the secondary effects of stopping the pill, should you experience any. It is generally all right to just stop the pill. Ask the doctor who prescribed it if it is fine to just stop. I recommend taking an herbal hormone supplement for one to two months before stopping the use of the pill if you have been taking it for five or more years. Vata women may need this supplement after only one year of use.

After stopping medication of any kind, the liver and kidneys should be strengthened for several months. The long-term use of pharmaceuticals damages these filters of the body, disturbs vata, and generally makes for long-term toxic accumulations in the digestive tract. Using a liver-cleansing formula is a good idea.

After this, it is best to take an immunemodulator (this supports immune function even after you stop taking it) for three months or more. These are the ones I suggest:

Vata: Use ashwagandha (2 gr.), shatavari (1 gr.), and triphala (1 gr.), twice a day with raw milk[1] and honey (8 grs. total per day)

Pitta: Use shatavari (2 gr), ashwagandha (1 gr.), and amla (1 gr.), twice a day with raw milk and raw sugar (8 grs total per day)

Kapha: Use ashwagandha (2 grs.), shatavari (1 gr.), and triphala (1 gr.), twice a day with warm water and honey (8 grs. total per day)

---

[1] Raw milk may be substituted with soya, rice, or almond milk, but they should always be warmed before taking.

Appendix 2

Pregnancy and Childbirth According to Ayurveda

This subject is worth a book in itself. In fact, the main text of ancient Ayurveda, the *Caraka Samhita*, spends about one-fourth of its many hundreds of pages just on women's health pertaining to childbirth. Despite the fact that I cannot address the topic in depth, not to mention it would be incorrect. So here I give a brief description of the Ayurvedic point of view of childbirth.

The most important thing is to be healthy *before* becoming pregnant. This means health according to Ayurveda, not just the absence of disease symptoms. There should be no toxins present in the body and the digestive system should be running smoothly. Menstruation should be smooth and without irregularities. Any irregularities in menstruation—pain, mood swings, excessive or minimal flow, irregular times of the cycle, or bloating and heaviness—will tend to give problems during both pregnancy and birthing. Your state before and during pregnancy will determine the actual birthing process. The healthier you are, the smoother the birth will be.

Ayurveda therefore stresses that you should be in good health before thinking of having children. This not only provides the baby a better chance to be born healthy, it also makes for an easier pregnancy and delivery. However, if you have become pregnant and you now want to improve your health, this can and should be done immediately. This involves the same steps outlined below, with the exception that the body should be mildly detoxified while strengthening it.

No drastic diets or regimes should be done during pregnancy by anyone. Nor should any recreational drugs be used at all—even tobacco or alcohol.

Ayurveda states that your state during pregnancy will influence the mind and body of the child. Obviously, this knowledge has been lost and disregarded by industrialized society for many generations—which may indicate why we have so many social problems today. Traditionally, a woman was cared for and nourished in mind, and in spirit, emotionally and physically. Emphasis was given to her emotional happiness and her contentment, because this was considered to be the greatest influence on the developing baby. Pregnant women were not allowed to work out of the home or be exposed to stress and combative environments. All of these factors disturb the developing child.

In today's world, we may not be able to follow these guidelines completely. We can, however, provide a loving environment and loving care to our pregnant friends, sisters, and relatives. Their husbands should be educated (admittedly, a difficult task) about the effects of childish jealousies and selfish needs on their spouses during pregnancy. They should support their partner in the creation of a new life. The pregnant woman, on the other hand, must nourish herself and her husband and family, because she is (whether anyone likes it or not) the pillar of the family. It is the feminine energy that holds everything together and provides the cohesion needed for a strong emotional base at home. Decidedly, woman must also be getting nourished to perform this increasingly difficult task.

The basic treatment is to strengthen and nourish the whole body. Care must be given to each tissue level, making sure that each system is working well throughout pregnancy. Mild exercises should be done. Hatha yoga for pregnant mothers is especially good, because it keeps the prana flowing smoothly though the body. This not only helps the child, but also makes for a much easier birthing. Diet is one of the most important factors and should be approached with care. Again, most books counsel high-protein diets, saying that protein builds the cell-wall structure in the body. Once more, it must be emphasized that modern researchers have repeatedly tried to make a diet that did not have enough protein and have failed every time. The only exception to this occurred when the diet was constructed of junk and processed foods. As long as you are eating foods in their natural state, you will get more than enough protein. By the same token, excessive amounts of protein may bring many problems for both yourself and your child.

Vitamins and supplements should also be approached with care. Taking supplements is rarely advised during pregnancy. If you are taking them, you should stop regularly to allow your body and baby a break. See chapter 6 if you are in doubt about this approach.

Even many herbs are contraindicated during pregnancy and these should also be used with caution. There are several exceptions. One of them is shatavari. Care should be used if you are kapha in constitution or have a tendency to bloat and gain weight, because shatavari will help to nourish you to such a degree that it can congest kapha types. Ayurveda considers ashwagandha to be good food during pregnancy. This view is not shared, however, in the West.

It goes without saying that, after birth, the child should be nursed for several months. This imparts so many nutrients that it is hard to comprehend why anyone would give a manufactured powder to a baby. More important still is the love which is passed from the mother to the child. Interfering with this time of bonding is one of the main problems in our society. Moreover, I have observed, over many years, that people who have not been breast fed are far more prone to allergies and food sensitivities.

All of pregnancy and childcare should be guided by a local professional and is too individual to merit general recommendations. This is one of the most important events in a woman's life and great care should be taken to support this event. The one common treatment advice that can be given is to love and be loved. This alone is enough to make up for many physical "shortcomings" and is the best cure for all neuroses. In Ayurveda, love itself is the most important treatment for pregnancy and the birth of a new being into this world.

Appendix 3

Aphrodisiacs and Fertility

As stated in chapter 4, there are three reasons why the humors go out of balance and cause disease: overstimulation of the senses and how we relate to the world through them; ignorance or a "failure of wisdom," which involves our habits, style of living, diet, and daily activities; and time. All three play a role in the fertility of a woman.

Medically, aphrodisiacs are substances that nourish the reproductive organs. They are not substances that stimulate a person to sexual excitement. The best aphrodisiac, in terms of sexual stimulation, is love. If you are looking for sexual excitement, this is the wrong book and the wrong appendix. Ayurveda has a whole science of aphrodisiacs. It is one of the eight branches of the medical system. It promotes healthy women, pregnancy, childbirth, and children.

Fertility and infertility relate directly to the seventh tissue level of the body. Any deficiency in this level of the body can result in low fertility. The science of aphrodisiacs in Ayurveda is the science of fertility.

The first important factor in fertility is the proper use of your sense organs. The vagina is a sense organ, the abuse of which affects the seventh tissue level of shukra. The mind is also a very subtle sense organ, the abuse of which will deplete the shukra. We can surmise that a history of abuse, sexually or mentally, can affect fertility. Being in a relationship that has no love can also disturb the shukra tissues. These factors must be addressed before taking aphrodisiacs and having success.

The second factor is perhaps the most important, because it covers everything we do in our lives. The shukra tissue level is, as mentioned before, the result of the other tissues. Lack of fertility usually shows a deficiency in all the tissues to some extent—mostly from a devitalized diet of junk or unnatural foods. Any action or habit that lessens the strength of the body or mind falls under this category and must be addressed before treatment.

The last factor is time, reflected in the movement of the doshas through the seasons and through the life. There is a very precise science that deals with time in the Vedic tradition and it is intimately linked with Ayurveda. This science is called *Jyotish*, or the "science of light." Light has always been the fundamental unit of time's movement for humans. In this sense, Jyotish can be used to find the best moment for fertility by observing the Moon. Jyotish is a very ancient system of lunar-based (feminine) astrology. Ayurvedic doctors never treat women for fertility without either consulting a Jyothisha or doing the birthchart themselves.

An understanding of time also indicates karmic factors, like the health of your mother or genetic problems. These show up in the birthchart. This is a special study in Jyotish and I am not trained in it, so I cannot offer any advice. However, there is an association in the United States that promotes this ancient knowledge and provides a list of qualified practitioners on request.[1] I suggest that, if fertility is a problem, you consult this association and find a practitioner in your area. By understanding your chart and the movement of the Moon through your life, you can identify the best moments to conceive. This should be done with the treatment advice I give below. It is a valid science, used successfully for many thousands of years. I use it medically in my own practice to help understand the movement of disease through time or to estimate the possible occurrence of disease in a patient's life.

To balance all three factors that disrupt the doshas, herbs and foods can be used. Before using the aphrodisiac

---

[1] Contact the American Council of Vedic Astrology at: P.O. Box 2149, Sedona, AZ 86339, Phone: (520) 282-6595, Fax: (520) 282-6097, acva@sedona.net.

herbs, you must have a clean system. If the body is not clean, the results will be mixed or the treatment may fail. If the body is too weak to clean itself, both cleansing and nourishing herbs should be used. The best aphrodisiac herbs in Ayurveda, in order of importance, are:

Shatavari
Ashwagandha
Shilajit
Lotus seeds
Amla
Dong quai
Gokshura
Guduchi
Bala

These herbs should be taken in doses of 4 to 8 grams a day in warm milk or water and with raw, natural sugar or honey. Ghee can also be used for pitta types or those with low agni.

Appendix 4

Herb Glossary

European and North American Herbs

English	Latin	Energies	Dosha
Agnus Castus	Vitex angnus castus	heating	vk-p+
Aloe gel	Aloe vulgaris	cooling	vpk=
Angelica	Angelica archangelica	heating	vk-p+
Ashwagandha	Withania somnifera	heating	vk-p+
Asparagus	Asparagus officialis	cooling	pk-v=
Barberry	Berberis vulgaris	heating	pk-v+
Bearberry—uva ursi	Arctostaphylos uva ursi	cooling	pk-v+
Black cohosh	Cimicifuga racemosa	cooling	pk-v+
Black haw	Viburnum punifolium	cooling	kv-p+
Borage	Borrago officinalis	cooling	pk-v+
Burdock	Arctium lappa	cooling	pk-v+
Calamus	Acorus calamus	heating	vk-p+
Calendula	Calendula officinalis	cooling	pk-p+
Cardamom	Elettaria cardamomum	heating	vk-p+
Chaste berries	Vitex agnus castus	heating	vk-p+
Chrysanthemum	Chrysanthemum morifolium	cooling	pk-v+
Cinnamon	Cinnamomum zeylanicum	heating	vk-p+
Comfrey	Symphyum officinale	cooling	pv-k+
Coriander	Coriandrum sativum	cooling	pkv=
Cramp bark	Viburnum opulus	heating	kv-p+
Cumin	Cuminum xanthorrhiza	cooling	pkv=
Dandelion	Taraxacum dens lenonis	cooling	pk-v+
Dong quai	Angelica sinensis	heating	vk-p=
Echinacea	Echinacea angustifolia	cooling	pk-v+
Elecampane	Inula helinium	heating	vk-p+
European madder	Rubia tinctorum	cooling	pk-v+
Fennel	Foeniculum vulgare	cooling	vpk=
Fenugreek	Trigonella foeniculum	heating	vk-p+
Gentian	Gentiana lutea	cooling	pk-v+
Ginger	Zingiber officinale	heating	vk-p+
Ginseng	Panax ginseng	heating	v-kp=

European and North American Herbs (cont.)

ENGLISH	LATIN	ENERGIES	DOSHA
Golden seal	Hydrastis canadensis	cooling	pk-v+
Gotu kola	Hydrocotyle asiatica	cooling	kpv=
Hawthorn berries	Crataegus oxyacantha	heating	v-k=p+
Licorice	Glycyrrhiza glabra	cooling	vp-k+
Marshmallow	Althaea officinalis	cooling	pv-k+
Mugwort	Artemesia vulgaris	heating	kv-p+
Myrrh	Commiphora myrrha	heating	kv-p+
Nettels	Urtica dioica	cooling	pk-v+
Nutmeg	Myristica fragans	heating	vk-p+
Raspberry	Rubus idoeus	cooling	pk-v+
Pennyroyal	Mentha pulegium	heating	vk-p+
Saffron	Crocus sativus	cooling	vpk=
Sage	Salvia officinalis	heating	kv-p+
Shatavari	Asparagus racemosus	cooling	pv-k+
Shepherd's purse	Capsella bursapastoris	cooling	pk-v+
St. John's Wort	Hypericum perforatum	cooling	pk-v+
Turmeric	Curcuma longa	heating	kv-p=
Valerian	Valeriana officinalis	heating	vk-p+
Yarrow	Achillea millefolium	cooling	pk-v-

Indian Herbs Alphabetically by English Names

English	Indian	Latin
Amrita	Guduchi	Tinispora cordifolia
Asafoetida	Hing	Asafoetida
Asparagus	Shatavari	Asparagus racemosus
Bamboo manna	Vamsha rochana	Bambusa arundinacia
Beleric myrobalan	Bibhitaki	Terminalia belerica
Black cumin	Kali jerra	Nigella sativa
Black pepper	Kalimirch	Piper nigrum
Calamus	Vacha	Acora calamus
Caltrops	Gokshura	Tribulis terrestris
Cardamom	Elacihi	Ellataria cardamomum
Castor bean or oil	Eranda	Ricinus communis
Ceylon leadwort	Chitrak	Plumbago zeylanica
Chebulic myrobalan	Haritaki	Terminalia chebula
Cinnamon	Dalchini	Cinnamomum zeylanicum
Clove	Lavanga	Caryophyllus aromaticus
Coriander	dhanyaka	Coriandrum sativum
Country mallow	bala	Sida cordifolia
Cowhage	Kaunch	Mucuna pruriens
Eclipta	Bhringraj	Eclipta alba
Embelia	Vidanga	Embelia ribes
Fennel	Bari saunf	Foeniculum vulgare
Ginger	Sunthi	Zingiber officinale
Gotu kola	Brahmi	Hydrocotyle asiatica
Guggulu	Guggulu	Commiphora mukul
Hog weed	Punarnava	Boerhaavia diffusa
Holy basil	Tulsi	Ocimum sanctum
Indian gentian	Chiraita	Swertia chirata
Indian gooseberry	Amal	Emblica officinalis
Indian madder	Manjishta	Rubia cordifolia
Indian sarsaparilla	Anantmool	Hemidesmus indicus
Indian valerian	Thagara	Valeriana wallichi
Licorice	Mulethi	Glycyrrhiza glabra
Lotus seeds	Kamal bees	Nelumbo nucifera
Long pepper	Pippli	Piper longum
Mineral pitch	Shilajit	Asphaltum
Neem	Neem	Azadiracta indica
Nut grass	Musta	Cyperus rotundus
Nutmeg	Jaiphal	Myristica fragrans
Picrorrhiza	Kutki	Picrorrhiza kurroa

Indian Herbs Alphabetically by English Names (cont.)

ENGLISH	INDIAN	LATIN
Saffron	Kesar	Crocus sativus
Sandalwood	Chandana	Santalum alba
Sesame	Tila	Sesamun indicum
Shankpushpi	Shankpushpi	Convolvolos pluricaulis
Solomon seal	Meda	Polygonatum officinale
Spikenard	Jatamansi	Nardostachys jatamansi
Tamala	Tejpatra	Cinnamomum iners
Turmeric	Haldi	Curcuma longa
White asparagus	Safed mushali	Asparagus adescendens
White cumin	Safed jerra	Cumimum cyminum
Winter cherry	Ashwagandha	Withania somnifera
Wood turmeric	Daru haldi	Berberis aristata

Appendix 5

Resources

Here are some resources for Ayurveda in the United States. The author has no affiliation with the products or services offered below. He is a certified teacher in Ayurveda for the American Institute of Vedic Studies in Europe.

Schools or Treatment Centers

American Institute of
    Vedic Studies
P.O. Box 8357
Santa Fe, NM 87504-8357
Tel: (505) 983-9385
Fax: (505) 982-5807
Email: vedicinst@aol.com
www.vedanet.com

The Ayurvedic Institute
P.O. Box 23445
Albuquerque, NM 87192-1445
Tel: (505) 291-9698
Fax: (505) 294-7572
www.ayurveda.com

California College for
    Ayurveda
1117-A East Main St.
Grass Valley, CA 95945
Tel: (530) 274-9100
Email:
info@ayurvedacollege.com
www.ayurvedacollege.com

The Chopra Center for
    Well-Being
7590 Fay Ave, Suite 403
LaJolla, CA 92037
Tel: (888) 424-6772
Fax: (619) 551-7825
www.CHOPRA.COM

New England Institute of
    Ayurvedic Medicine
111 N. Elm St., Suites 103–105
Worcester, MA 01609
Tel: (508) 755-3744
Fax: (508) 770-0618
Email:
AYURVEDA@HOTMAIL.COM
www.GIS.NET/~AYURVEDA

Wise Earth School of
    Ayurveda
(A nonprofit organization)
Rte. 1 Box 484
Chandler, NC 28715
Tel: (828) 258-9999

Vinayak Ayurveda Center
2509 Virginia NE, Suite D
Albuquerque, NM 87110
Tel: (505) 296-6522
Fax: (505) 298-2932

Herbal Suppliers

The Ayurvedic Institute
P.O. Box 23445
Albuquerque, NM 87192-
1445
Tel: (505) 291-9698
Fax: (505) 294-7572
www.ayurveda.com

Banyan Trading Co.
P.O. Box 13002
Albuquerque, NM 87192
Tel: (800) 953-6424
      (505) 244-1880
Fax: (505) 244-1878
www.BANYANTRADING.COM

Bazaar of India Imports, Inc.
1810 University Ave.
Berkeley, CA 94703
Tel: (800) 261-7662

BioVeda
215 North Route 303
Congers, NY 10920
Tel: (800) 292-6002

Dhanvantri Aushadhalaya
P.O. Box 1654
San Anselmo, CA 94979
Tel: (415) 289-7976
www.dhanvantri.com

Internatural
33719 116th Street
Box AH
Twin Lakes, WI 53181
Tel: (800) 643-4221
Fax: (414) 889-8591
Email:
internatural@lotuspress.com
www.internatural.com

Sushakti
1840 Iron St., Suite C
Bellingham, WA 98225
Tel: (888) 774-2584
Tel: (360) 752-0575
Email: info@ayurveda-
sushakti.com
www.ayurveda-sushakti.com

Vinayak Ayurveda Center
2509 Virginia NE, Suite D
Albuquerque, NM 87110
Tel: (505) 296-6522
Fax: (505) 298-2932

Information on Herbs

The Herb Research Foundation
1007 Pearl St. Suite 200
Boulder, CO 80302
Tel: (303) 449-2265
Fax: (303) 449-7849
Email: info@herbs.org
www.herbs.org

This is a nonprofit organization that publishes research articles on over 200 different plants. They also have a good report on herb safety. Some of the research for this book and others that I have written has come from this organization. Their point of view is basically biochemical. Recommended.

Glossary

abhyanga: therapeutic or daily massage.

agni: first of three cosmic principles; god of fire; digestive fire.

allopathy: Western medicine, modern medicine.

apana prana: one of the five pranas; the prana that controls all evacuation, called the downward breath; resides in the lower abdomen.

aphrodisiac: any substance that promotes health to the reproductive organs.

ashram: place devoted to spiritual development.

astanga hrdayam: one of the three ancient Ayurvedic texts of medicine.

atma: consciousness or God in an individualized sense.

Ayurveda: oldest medical system in the world; a holistic approach developed by the same sages who formed the systems of yoga; part of the Vedas dealing with the health of the body; the science of life.

brimhana: strengthening or fortifying therapies in Ayurveda.

brahma: consciousness in an absolute sense; one of the three aspects of consiousness, the creator or creative aspect; the founder of Ayurveda in the form of a god.

brahman: term used to describe that which it is not possible to describe; often just called being, conscious, bliss, or sat, chit, anand; the Self.

brahmin: the learned class of people in Vedic society; priests.

bramhacharya: abidance in Brahma or the unmanifest reality; often incorrectly used to mean forced celibacy.

Caraka Samhita: the oldest surviving text of Ayurveda; one of the three ancient Ayurvedic texts of medicine.

chi: Chinese word for prana.

chit: consciousness.

consciousness: as used in this book, the substratum or source of all manifestation.

constitution: an individual's unique mix of the three humors.

dhatu: tissue; there are seven different tissue levels in Ayurveda—plasma, blood, muscle, fat, bone, bone marrow and nerve tissue, and reproductive fluids.

dosha: Sanskrit for "humor"; literally, that which will imbalance or go out; "fault."

energetic impressions: in Sanskrit there are two kinds, vasanas and samskaras; latent, unconscious, or stored impressions and current mental impressions; impressions stored in the subtle body; yoga says that these impressions are what cause us to incarnate in another life, unless they are allowed to surface to consciousness; these impressions, along with prana, create what we call mind.

inquiry: method to find out where thoughts, prana arise; question: "Who am I?" (see books of Ramana Maharishi and H. W. L. Poonjaji).

five elements: the five states of material existence: mass, liquidity, transformation, movement, and the field in which they function; also called: earth, water, fire, air, and ether.

five states of matter: commonly called the Five Elements.

ghee: butter that has gone through a process of cooking to render it free from deterioration; used for cooking and as a vehicle for herbal medicines.

guna: quality, attribute of intelligence; there are three gunas: sattva, rajas, and tamas; therapeutically there are twenty that determine the quality of herb or substance (i.e., oily, slimy, dry, etc.).

guru: literally "dispeller of ignorance"; one who knows the substratum or source of creation; teacher; heavy.

humor: a unique concept to describe the functions of the body; the forces that balance the five elements together in the body; there are three humors: vata (wind), pitta (fire), and kapha (water). There is a fourth humor called the "sense of humor" which is often lacking in people, but is worthwhile to develop.

kapha: one of the three humors; that which binds; cohesion; controls water and earth elements.

karma: action; the cosmic law that for every action there is a reaction; there is no such thing as "bad or good" karma; therapeutically, the general action of an herb or substance in the body.

ki: Japanese word for prana.

kundalini: the primordial prana that rests dormant in the body unless activated by special practices (note: these practices are dangerous unless one is supervised by a *qualified* teacher).

langhana: reducing therapies in Ayurveda.

latent impression: see *energetic impressions.*

life force: another name for prana, especially those five vayus in the body.

mantra: the science of sound; by using the correct sound, each prana can be harmonized—and so the mind.

marma: a sensitive point on the body that stimulates the pranic flow; the acupressure points of Ayurveda.

maya: the illusion that everything exists as separate from God.

meridians: the channels of prana in the body; called nadis in yoga and the prana srota in Ayurveda.

mind: thoughts moving through consciousness, giving the illusion of continuity; the combination of prana and vasanas.

nadi: see *meridian.*

ojas: the essence of food and the outcome of the seventh tissue level; the basis of the immune system. We are born with eight drops of ojas in the heart center. If this is reduced, death results. There is a secondary ojas which is the result of all the tissue elements. It can vary in quantity, however, when it is reduced, sickness results (see Caraka Samhita, vol. I, p. 594).

pancha karma: the Five Actions; five reducing therapies in Ayurveda.

parabdha: the karma or action that is residual; the karmas associated with the body/mind manifestation. In other words, as long as you have a body, the parabdha karma continues.

pitta: one of the three humors; that which burns; transformation; controls fire and water elements.

prakriti: the dynamic energy of consciousness; Mother Nature; natal constitution.

prana: pra = before, ana = breath; vayu; the vital force; Qi, Ki, Chi; arises from substratum of pure consciousness with intelligence (agni) and love (soma). Together they create the individualized consciousness. There are five major pranas in the human body, prana, apana, samana, udana, and vyana. They arise from the cosmic prana and the rajas guna; chief of the five vayus in the body, called the outward-going breath, it resides in the head and the heart.

pranayama: method of breath control used to regulate the mind and the prana, and thereby physical and mental health; should only be practiced with a *qualified* teacher.

pranic healing: a therapeutic method that harmonizes the pranas directly.

purusha: unmanifest aspect of consciousness; the void; pure intelligence; masculine energy.

qi: another name for prana.

rajas: one of the three gunas; action, movement, bright, energy, aggression, aggravated mind, achievement, and strong emotions.

samana prana: one of the five pranas in the body; called the equalizing prana; resides in the navel region.

samsara: concept that we are separate from God; suffering; illusion.

samskaras: innate or conditioned energetic impressions; see *energetic impressions.*

sattva: one of the three gunas; purity, peace, calm, beauty, happiness, quiet obedient mind, and stable emotions.

sattvic diet: a diet that promotes sattva; very mild nourishing foods like milk, basmati rice, mung beans, and fruits.

Self: another name for pure consciousness; also called Brahman, or the substratum of all duality—i.e., creation; our true nature, hence the term "Self"; sometimes given as "I-I" in Indian books.

Shakti: or Sakti; cosmic prana; the wife of Shiva; the dynamic aspect of feminine energy.

Shiva: or Siva; pure consciousness; one of the three aspects of consciousness as god, the destroyer.

snehana: massage using oils as part of oleation therapy; generally used as preparation for pancha karma.

soma: nectar; the most subtle essence of ojas and kapha; the god Soma signifies love, unity.

srotas: channels in the Ayurvedic system that carry substances like blood, air, and thought.

substratum: equal to The Absolute, pure Consciousness, Love, Brahman, Atman, Self, or Source.

Sushruta Samhita: one of the three ancient Ayurvedic texts of medicine.

tamas: one of the three gunas; inertia, dull, depressed, void, stupid, lazy, despair, and self-destructive emotions.

tantra: A path that totally accepts all aspects of the physical world, believing that all things lead to the divine; worship of the divine mother; often confused with sexual practice.

taste: the beginning of the therapeutic actions of any substance on the body.

tejas: the subtle form of pitta; the power of discrimination in the mind.

trikutu: a famous Ayurvedic formula that stimulates digestion and agni; very good for kapha.

triphala: a famous Ayurvedic formula for rejuvenating the body, promoting digestion, and harmonizing all the digestive organs; good for all three humors.

udana prana: one of the five pranas in the body; called the upward-moving breath, it is seated in the throat; kundalini yoga cultivates this prana, as do all psychic powers.

vasanas: latent energetic impression, see *energetic impressions.*

vata: one of the three humors; that which blows; movement; controls wind (air) and ether elements.

Vayu: the God of the Wind; another name for vata; another name for prana.

Vedas: literally, "knowledge", but used here to mean the Book of Knowledge, the oldest book in the world; there are four Vedas.

vikruti: the constitution of the moment; that which covers prakruti.

vishnu: consciousness as pure love; the aspect of consciousness that protects and preserves the world; as a god, Vishnu has seven main manifestations, of which Rama and Krishna are the two most famous.

vyana prana: one of the five pranas in the body; called the equalizing breath, it unifies all the other pranas and the body, it is defused throughout the body.

yantra: a sound or syllable transformed into a geometric form, usually inscribed in a metal plate or in stone.

yoga: union; that which leads one back to the original Source; generally understood to mean a path or a practice leading to the Divine; not limited to hatha yoga or asanas.

Bibliography

Astanga Hrdayam. vols. I–III. Prof. K. R. Srikantha Murthy, trans. Varanasi, India: Krishnadas Academy, 3rd ed., 1996.

Atreya. *Practical Ayurveda: Secrets of Physical, Sexual & Spiritual Health*. York Beach, ME: Samuel Weiser, 1998.

———. *Prana: The Secret of Yogic Healing*. York Beach, ME: Samuel Weiser, 1996.

———. *The Secrets of Ayurvedic Massage*. Twin Lakes, WI: Lotus Press, 1999.

Ballentine, Dr. Rudolph. *Diet and Nutrition: A Holistic Approach*. Honesdale, PA: Himalayan International Institute, 1978.

Chen, Junshi, et al. *Diet, Lifestyle, and Mortality in China: A Study of the Characteristics of 65 Countries*. T. C. Campbell, et al. eds. Ithaca, NY: Cornell University Press, 1990.

Clifford, Terry. *Tibetan Buddhist Medicine and Psychiatry*. York Beach, ME: Samuel Weiser, 1984.

Dash, Dr. Bhagwan. *Ayurvedic Cures for Common Diseases*. 4th ed. Delhi, India: Hind Pocket Books, 1993.

Dash, Dr. Bhagwan, and Dr. R. K. Sharma. *Caraka Samhita*. 3 vols. Varanasi, India: Chowkamba Series Office, 1992.

Devaraj, Dr. T. L. *Speaking of Ayurvedic Remedies for Common Diseases*, New Delhi, India: Sterling Publishers, 1985.

Frawley, Dr. David. *Astrology of the Seers*. Twin Lakes, WI: Lotus Press 2000.

———. *Ayurveda and the Mind: The Healing of Consciousness*. Twin Lakes, WI: Lotus Press, 1997.

———. *Ayurvedic Healing: A Comprehensive Guide*. Twin Lakes, WI: Lotus Press 2000.

————. *Gods, Sages and Kings: Vedic Secrets of Ancient Civilization.* Twin Lakes, WI: Lotus Press 1991.

————. *Tantric Yoga and the Wisdom Goddesses.*   Twin Lakes, WI: Lotus Press 2003.

Frawley, Dr. David, and Dr. Vasant Lad. *The Yoga of Herbs.* Twin Lakes, WI: Lotus Press, 1986.

Grieve, Mrs. M. *A Modern Herbal.* London: Tiger Books International, rev. ed., 1973.

Heyn, Birgit. *Ayurvedic Medicine: The Gentle Strength of Indian Healing.* New Delhi, India: Indus/Harper-Collins India, 1992.

Joshi, Dr. Sunil V. *Ayurveda and Panchakarma.* Twin Lakes, WI: Lotus Press, 1996.

Lad, Dr. Vasant. *Ayurveda: The Science of Self-Healing.* Twin Lakes, WI: Lotus Press, 1984.

————. *Secrets of the Pulse.* Albuquerque, NM: The Ayurvedic Institute, 1996.

Lad, Dr. Vasant, and Usha Lad. *Ayurvedic Cooking for Self-Healing.* Twin Lakes, WI: Lotus Press, 1994.

Lee, John R., and Virginia Hopkins. *What Your Doctor May Not Tell You about Menopause: The Breakthrough Book on Natural Progesterone.* New York: Warner, 1996.

Miller, Dr. Light, and Dr. Bryan Miller. *Ayurveda and Aromatherapy.* Twin Lakes, WI: Lotus Press, 1995.

Morningstar, Amadea. *The Ayurvedic Cookbook.* Twin Lakes, WI: Lotus Press, 1990.

————. *Ayurvedic Cooking for Westerners.* Twin Lakes, WI: Lotus Press, 1994.

Nisargadatta, Maharaj. *Consciousness and the Absolute.* Durham, NC: Acorn Press, 1994.

————. *I Am That.* Bombay, India: Chetana Ltd., 1991.

————. *Prior to Consciousness* Durham. NC: Acorn Press, 1985.

————. *Seeds of Consciousness.* Durham, NC: Acorn Press, 1990.

Poonja, Sri H. W. L. *Papaji*. David Godman, ed., Boulder, CO: Avadhuta Foundation, 1993.

———. *The Truth Is.* San Anselmo, CA: Vidya Sagar Publications, 1995.

———. *Wake Up and Roar*, vols. I & II. Kula, Maui, Hawaii: Pacific Center Pub., 1992.

Ramana Maharishi. *Be As You Are*. David Godman, ed., New Delhi, India: Penguin Books India, 1992.

———. *Talks With Sri Ramana Maharishi*. Swami Ramanananda, trans. Tiruvannamalai, India: Sri Ramanasramam, 1984.

Ramanananda, Swami, trans. *Advaita Bodha Deepika*. Tiruvannamalai, India: Sri Ramanasramam, 1990.

———. trans. *Tripura Rahasya*. Tiruvannamalai, India: Sri Ramanasramam, 1989.

Ranade, Dr. Subhash & Frawley, David. *Ayurveda: Natures Medicine.* Twin Lakes, WI: Lotus Press 2003.

Robbins, John. *Diet for a New America*, Walpole, NH: Stillpoint Publishing, 1987.

———. *Diet for a New World*. New York: Avon Books, 1992.

Rogers, Carol. *The Women's Guide to Herbal Medicine*. London: Hamish Hamilton, 1995.

Ros, Dr. Frank. *The Lost Secrets of Ayurvedic Acupuncture*. Twin Lakes, WI: Lotus Press, 1994.

Sachs, Melanie. *Ayurvedic Beauty Care*. Lotus Press, WI: Twin Lakes, 1994.

Sharma, Dr. Priya Vrat. *Sodasangahrdayam—Essentials of Ayurveda*. Delhi, India: Motilal Banarsidass Publishers, 1993.

Svoboda, Dr. Robert. *Ayurveda: Life, Health and Longevity*. New Delhi, India: Penguin/Books India, 1993.

———. *Prakruti: Your Ayurvedic Constitution*. Twin Lakes, WI: Lotus Press 1998.

Tierra, Michael. *Planetary Herbology*. Twin Lakes, WI: Lotus Press, 1988.

———. *The Way of Herbs*. New York: Pocket Books, 1998.

Tiwari, Maya. *Ayurveda: Secrets of Healing.* Twin Lakes, WI: Lotus Press, 1995.

Yoga Vasistha: The Supreme Yoga. vols. I & II. Swami Venkatesananda, trans. Shivanandanagar, Uttar Pradesh, India: Divine Life Society, 1991.

Weed, Susun S. *Breast Cancer? Breast Health! The Wise Woman Way.* Woodstock, NY: Ash Tree Publishing, 1996.

———. *Menopausal Years: The Wise Woman Way.* Woodstock, NY: Ash Tree Publishing, 1992.

———. *Wise Woman Herbal for the Childbearing Year.* Woodstock, NY: Ash Tree Publishing, 1986.

Index

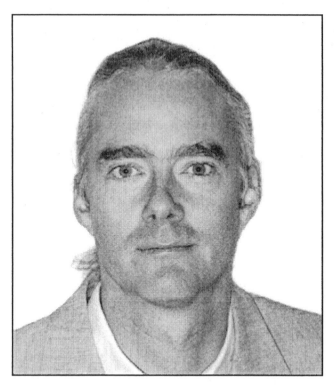

Atreya became interested in metaphysics and meditation at the age of 17. He lived in India for six years studying meditation, pranic healing, Ayurveda, and yogic physchology. He studied under Sri Ramana Maharishi's disciple, Sri H. W. L. Poonja, for several years and this experience completely changed his approach to the healing arts. Originally from Southern California, and after living in India, he now resides in France, where he practices Ayurvedic and pranic healing. Groups who want to arrange workshops or seminars are welcome to contact Atreya through the publisher. He is the author of Prana: The Secrets of Yogic Healing (Weiser, 1996) and Practical Ayurveda: Secrets for Physical, Sexual & Spiritual Health (Weiser, 1998); and Secrets of Ayurvedic Massage (Lotus Press, 1999).